Good Food, Good Mood

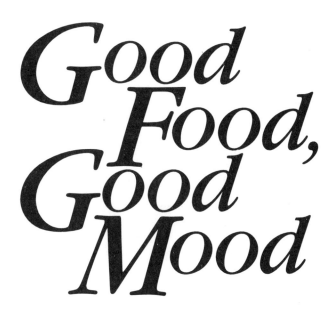

Good Food, Good Mood

Treating Your Hidden Allergies

GARY NULL
with
Dr. MARTIN FELDMAN

Dodd, Mead & Company
New York

No part of this book may be reproduced in any form
without permission in writing from the publisher.
Published by Dodd, Mead & Company, Inc.,
71 Fifth Ave. New York, N.Y. 10003
Manufactured in the United States of America
Designed by Elizabeth Frenchman
First Edition

    4 5 6 7 8 9 10

Library of Congress Cataloging-in-Publication Data

Null, Gary.
  Good food, good mood : treating your hidden allergies / by Gary
Null with Martin Feldman.—1st ed.
    p. cm.
  Bibliography: p.
  Includes index.
  1. Food allergy—Popular works. 2. Food allergy—Diet therapy—
Recipes. I. Feldman, Martin, 1939–   II. Title.
RC596.N85 1988
616.97′50654—dc19
ISBN 0-396-08981-X

                                                88–300
                                                CIP

Contents

Acknowledgments

Several hundred interviews were conducted to complete this book. Most of the leading clinical ecologists in the country were interviewed. All of those interviewed gave freely of their time, information, and research files. They include: Dr. Theron Randolph, Dr. Marshall Mandell, Dr. Doris Rapp, Dr. Janice Keller Phelps, Dr. William G. Crook, Dr. Michael B. Schacter, Dr. Richard Podell, Dr. Ray C. Wunderlich, Jr., Dr. Roy Kupsinel, Dr. William H. Philpott, and Dr. Karl E. Humiston, to name but a few.

In addition, I would like to give special thanks to Mary Ann Reidy, M.S., whose assistance was invaluable in synopsizing dozens of hours of taped interviews and hundreds of scientific research papers. I am also grateful to Judy Trupin, who helped research and edit text on several topics. Finally, I thank Martin Feldman, M.D., who acted as medical reviewer in the chapter on treatments. Dr. Feldman is affiliated with Mount Sinai Hospital in New York City.

This manuscript has gone through several stages to completion. At each stage I was assisted by my editor Julie Weiner, researcher Phil Hodes, Ph.D., and a very special associate, Trudy Golobic, Esq. Trudy worked several hundred hours, helping verify facts, restyling sections of the manuscript, and doing interviews. Lastly, this book was encouraged and motivated by one unique person: Robin Bartlett. Robin supported my efforts at every stage of this book. Many thanks, Robin.

Introduction

THE GREAT MASQUERADER

Do you or does anyone you know suffer from arthritis? Migraine? Chronic fatigue? Mental illness? There is a chance that these disorders are the symptoms of a food allergy – without your even knowing it.

For some people, recognizing allergies is simple. They sneeze when they are around a cat, or they develop hives immediately after eating strawberries. For others, allergies aren't so obvious.

Headaches, stomachaches, fatigue, depression, and even serious mental illness and criminal behavior can be caused by allergic response.

Those who suffer from the subtle allergy often follow a lonely path. They go from specialist to specialist, only to be told that their problems are emotionally rooted. Or worse, they may be treated with psychotherapy and drugs, when such costly treatments are irrelevant. Worse yet, they may be told there is nothing wrong at all.

For this reason, allergy has been called "the great masquerader."

THE ROLE OF THE CLINICAL ECOLOGIST

It's a shame that the cause of so much suffering should go unrecognized and hence untreated. Fortunately, today there is a new breed of physician who has broadened the definition of allergy.

These progressive practitioners are known as *clinical ecologists* or environmental medicine specialists. Because of their work, many previously unrecognized allergy sufferers are being successfully diagnosed and treated.

Clinical ecology is the subspecialty of environmental medicine that focuses on our interrelationship with the immediate environment. It is based on the principle that a person who is exposed to environmental chemicals – such as pesticides, food additives, and water and air pollutants affecting one's workplace or home (including gas fumes, molds, dust, animal danders, and so on) – may have adverse reactions to them. These reactions may cause a wide range of mental, emotional, and physical disorders in adults, children, and even pets.

Clinical ecologists use many of traditional allergists' techniques, as well as several they have created – such as sublingual provocative testing and intradermal neutralization therapy (discussed later on in this book) – and they take a detailed environmental history of the patient. In addition, they often prescribe rotational diets, which attempt to identify foods that are implicated in the patient's ailments. Eggs, wheat, corn, dairy products, sugar, yeast, and beef are the primary culprits.

Many clinical ecologists started out as traditional board-certified allergists, but found themselves frustrated because they weren't always able to help their patients by conventional means. They would often hear themselves telling patients that their chronic headaches, arthritis flare-ups, or mood swings were "just your imagination" or suggesting vague remedies like "reducing stress" and sending them home with a prescription for a mood-altering drug. Such discouraging experiences have led these practitioners to look more deeply into the nature and sources of allergy.

They have read the scientific literature written by such experts as Dr. Theron G. Randolph; Dr. William Rea; and Dr. William Kaufman. These pioneers, working with thousands of patients, have discovered, for instance, that in some cases they can turn a person's arthritis pain on and off with a tiny drop of extract of a specific allergen (e.g., corn, wheat, or egg) under the tongue.

Other members of the field have taken specific training sessions that include in-depth workshops, a three-part course, qualifying examinations, and extensive residency programs at special allergy hospitals, such as Brookhaven Hospital in Dallas, Texas, where Dr. Rea directs the Environmental Health Center. (Dr. Rea specializes in allergic reactions that affect the cardiovascular system.)

To keep the medical world as well as their colleagues informed of their research and their latest discoveries, clinical ecologists publish and contribute to *The Archives of Clinical Ecology*, a well-respected publication.

If you wish to consult with a clinical ecologist, you may obtain the names of those practicing in your area by writing to the American Academy of Environmental Medicine, P.O. Box 16106, Denver, Colorado 80216.

PREVIOUSLY UNAVAILABLE INFORMATION

One of the healthiest American obsessions is our need to define and challenge the ways in which we are being manipulated. We have an unquenchable thirst for asserting our freedom and seeking out the truth. For this reason readers will find the following fact disturbing: Much of the "new" knowledge concerning allergies has been around *for more than fifty years*, but it was not made available to the public!

This book will explain in detail why the truth has remained suppressed for so long.

A NEW APPROACH

Unlike traditional allergists, clinical ecologists do not rely on drug therapy to "combat" allergic reactions. Rather, they work closely with the patient to identify all harmful substances, however subtle their effects, and to root them out of the patient's life.

The clinical ecologist recognizes that an allergic response can occur in any human organ, including the stomach and the brain. He or she uses tests not performed by traditional allergists to pick up otherwise unidentified sensitivities.

When allergenic substances are removed from these patients' lives, they find relief from symptoms that have troubled them for years!

For those who suspect that their symptoms are allergy-related, this book offers valuable assistance in identifying problems and learning about treatments.

The case studies used in the book to exemplify specific symptoms, diagnoses, and treatments are based on true cases, although the names – and sometimes the personal circumstances – have been altered.

THE RECIPES

If you're an average American, your daily diet contains a frightening number of toxic chemicals. From the pesticides in our fruits and vegetables to the antibiotics and tranquilizers in our meat, Americans are slowly being poisoned.

Enumerated in the following pages are the many ways our chemical-ridden diet and environment adversely affect our health. Included as a healthful nutrition alternative, are dozens of delicious, high-protein recipes – as well as related dietary information – carefully designed to help keep your diet and your life freer of chemicals and of allergic reactions.

If you are interested in your health – and who isn't? – this book will teach you how to keep your body less toxic in an increasingly polluted world.

CHAPTER ONE

Recognizing Our Symptoms

HIDDEN FOOD ALLERGIES

CASE ONE* On one bright, sunny Sunday morning, eight-year-old Timmy Potter woke up in dismay. He had wet his bed again, as he did nearly every night. He quickly gathered the sheets together and, avoiding his mother, dragged them to the washing machine. When Mrs. Potter poked her head into Timmy's room to see if he was awake, the stripped bed stared at her. *Not again,* she thought.

Timmy's mother felt nagging and unbearable doubt that she and her husband were somehow failing Timmy. They decided right then and there that her son's "accidents" had gone on long enough. First thing Monday morning she made an appointment for Timmy with a urologist and, after giving it some thought, another appointment – with a psychiatrist.

Timmy's already high levels of frustration, embarrassment, and anxiety were increased by the mental and physical probing first of his parents and then of his doctors at these and other appointments. He began to misbehave at home and at school. Soon teachers and physicians labeled him a neurotic child with a behavior problem. No one suspected that Timmy's problem was a physiological reaction to something in his diet.

---

*All the case studies in this book are based on true accounts reported by clinical ecologists. The patients' names have been changed to protect their privacy.

Fortunately for Timmy, one of his teachers called his mother and asked if Timmy had ever been tested for food allergies. The teacher told Mrs. Potter that several children in her classes had literally been transformed when certain foods were eliminated from their diets. Timmy's mother was skeptical, but she jotted down the name of the pediatric allergist that the teacher recommended and made an appointment for Timmy the next week.

After following for a week the restricted diet that the doctor recommended, Timmy seemed better. He hadn't wet his bed, he seemed more cooperative and in a better mood, and he seemed to understand his homework better. But Mrs. Potter was not convinced; maybe it was just wishful thinking.

The following week she took Timmy back for testing. Timmy was told by the physician to eat as much sugar as he wanted. Before her eyes, Mrs. Potter saw Timmy transform. By his eighth sugar cube, Timmy whined and pouted. He shoved things off of the table in front of him, and he wet his pants.

The doctor explained to Mrs. Potter that this was not that unusual; that many children who are diagnosed as hyperactive, learning disabled, or just plain neurotic are, in fact, simply allergic to some of the foods they commonly eat. In Timmy's case the food was cane sugar.

At first, Mrs. Potter found that keeping Timmy on a sugar-free diet was not easy. Sugar was in his cereal, in bread, in catsup—in fact, it was in almost every prepared or packaged food that he ate. She experimented with products from her local health-food store, but sometimes she was lax. Whenever that happened, or when Timmy binged on cakes or cookies after school, he reverted back to his old self. Each time this happened, Mrs. Potter's resolve grew stronger. Finally, after a year or so, it was second nature for both Timmy and Mrs. Potter to buy only dried fruits or fruit-juice-sweetened cookies for dessert and to use maple syrup, date sugar, or rice syrup as a sweetener.

Today Timmy no longer wets his bed. He is a good student in school and generally is a good, "normal" kid.

CASE TWO   Angela was in her midthirties and had three children. She was obsessed with cleaning, and she felt an odd sense of domestic adventure when she experimented with new household products. But Angela was not as healthy as she could be. Some days she had severe headaches, and on other days she experienced irrational mood swings, ranging from deep depression to violent anger.

Angela neglected the children when she was in one of her blue funks, and she abused them during her fits of anger. After the mood swings subsided, Angela hated herself for hurting her children. She began to doubt her sanity; she sought psychiatric help and was prescribed mood elevators and tranquilizers.

At first, no connection was made between Angela's erratic behavior and the cleaning agents she used so often. But as time went on, Tony, Angela's husband, began to worry about all the drugs the psychiatrist had prescribed for her. He decided to call a friend of his who had been raving about a nutritional doctor he was seeing. Tony thought the "health-food kick" that his friend was on was a lot of nonsense, but he had to admit his friend looked better than he had looked in years. Tony got the name of the doctor and made an appointment for Angela.

After about an hour of taking Angela's case history, the doctor told Angela that he suspected she was sensitive to some of the cleaning products she used since she was around them constantly. After testing, the doctor determined that Angela was, in fact, very allergic to chlorine bleach, which was present in both her bleach and her scouring powder. When she eliminated the bleach and bought a new, milder cleanser from a Shaklee distributor, her headaches and fits of anger went away, and her mood swings settled down.

ENVIRONMENTAL ALLERGIES

There is a common thread that weaves through these stories. The common thread is *environmental allergy*, a response to substances tolerated by most persons. Something in Timmy's, and Angela's food or environment had caused them to have a distressing physical or mental response, creating anxiety both for the sufferers and for those around them.

When Timmy and Angela sought help along traditional medical avenues, their symptoms were invalidated. Their psychological and physical problems were compounded by the doctors' skepticism that anything was legitimately "wrong." The reason for the doctors' disbelief was that their specific forms of allergy did not fall within the narrow definition of allergy used by conventional allergists.

In general, allergies are often mismanaged because the general public and many physicians don't know enough about their symptoms, approaches, and treatments. Clinical ecologists, recognizing this knowledge gap, have dedicated their practices to filling it.*

Ecology is the branch of science concerned with the interrelationships between organisms and their environment. The clinical ecologist keeps this interrelationship in mind when relieving allergic suffering. Unfortunately, wide acceptance of their applications and research has been held in check by prevailing allergy doctrine, which, as we shall see, is not always the most effective or the most scientifically sound.

Clinical ecologists, employing the principles of holistic medicine, care for the whole being, a being who is a single unit operating within its environment. Given a patient with a problem – say, a baby with severe colic – a conventional physician might treat it with a drug that suppresses the symptom rather than fully seeking the *source* of the symptom. A clinical ecologist, presented with the same baby, will *always* seek to find the *cause* of the colic. The aim is to remove the cause of illness from the baby's environment, in the expectation that the illness will then disappear.

TWO SCHOOLS OF THOUGHT

The study of allergies has had a volatile history. The term *allergy* is derived from the Greek for "altered reaction." It initially conveyed the idea that certain substances in the environment could evoke adverse reactions in some individuals while having no effect on the public at large. Early twentieth-century allergists readily acknowledged that a person is part of his or her environment. When an individual developed an otherwise unexplainable symptom, his or her food intake and surroundings were investigated for possible causes. Diagnosis and treatment supported the concept of environmental exposure.

---

*Clinical ecologists and their work are described more fully in the Introduction to this book.

Then around 1925 the majority of allergists began to restrict their definition of *allergy* to accord with what is called the "antigen-anti-body theory." According to this theory only those reactions that resulted in a *measurably* abnormal immune response to a particular substance (or allergen) were recognized as allergies by physicians. Acceptance of this theory coincided with the wide acceptance of the Ishizaka study, which proved that immunoglobin E (or IgE) contains human (detects allergies) reaginic antibody; it also coincides with scientific advances that made the detection and measurement of antibody levels even more precise. In this new, narrow definition of allergy, only an altered immune response constituted allergy.

While this new definition of allergy rendered the field eminently more scientific and hence more acceptable to the orthodox medical community, it also substantially limited the field. Today the traditional allergist (i.e., one practicing according to the antigen-antibody theory) on the whole will diagnose as an allergy only the most dramatic reactions, such as runny nose, sneezing, hives, and rashes. Most of these dramatic reactions are physical. Ignored by these traditional allergists are more subtle reactions to environmental substances that may not be accompanied by the altered immune response readily detectable by current technology. These subtle reactions can include a wide variety of altered mental, emotional, or behavioral states, such as hyperactivity, depression, fatigue, and schizophrenia.

The majority of allergists trained after 1925 accepted the immunological definition of allergy, which was taught them in the medical schools. This acceptance resulted in a marked "tunnel-vision" approach to allergy by orthodox practitioners; they denied clinically substantiated allergic phenomena that fell outside their definition. Yet a few specialists – the forerunners of clinical ecologists – found this definition too narrow. They preferred to practice according to the original definition of allergy, which was broad enough to encompass any "altered reaction" a particular individual might have to a particular substance in his or her environment.

Today, although there is some overlap, there still remain two distinct kinds of allergists. One is the traditional allergist, who in accordance with the antigen-antibody theory confines the diagnosis of allergy to immunoglobin E or other immune-mediated conditions.

Their primary method of treatment is the utilization of drugs to suppress symptoms. The other kind is the clinical ecologist, who, while recognizing IgE-mediated allergies, uses a wider definition of allergy. Their primary focus in treating allergies is on eliminating or neutralizing the cause of the allergy.

WHAT IS AN ALLERGY?

Traditional allergists and clinical ecologists say basically the same thing about allergy – namely, that it is an immune response to a foreign substance or *antigen*. The difference between them lies primarily in their clinical approach to allergy. The traditional allergist confines his or her diagnosis of allergy to those cases that present the recognized immune responses. The clinical ecologist, however, diagnoses allergy in a much larger number of cases, even though he or she may not be able to explain precisely the cause of an immune response. For instance, Doris Rapp, M.D., a professor of pediatrics at the State University of New York at Buffalo and author of *Allergies and the Hyperactive Child*, explains the nature of allergy essentially in terms of the antigen-antibody theory. However, Dr. Rapp and many other clinical ecologists readily admit that although they believe an immune response in the form of an antigen-antibody reaction is at the root of allergic reactions, they are not always able to explain how this occurs. It may be through IgE, IgG (an antibody produced by the B cell, an overabundance of which can cause mild perspiring to depression), or other immunoglobulins we have isolated, or it may occur in ways that we cannot yet scientifically detect.

Dr. Rapp explains how a defense reaction by your immune system can show up as an allergic reaction:

> An antigen is anything that is foreign to your body. It could be food, dust, pollen or cat hair. It is something that isn't part of you. It comes into the body and the body says, 'Hey! This is not normal.' The body forms a protection called an antibody.
>
> To make it very simple, there are good antibodies and bad antibodies. When a germ comes into your body and is joined by a good antibody, the antigen is neutralized so that you don't have any trouble with that particular organism and you don't get sick.

When you have an allergy, you eat a food or drink a liquid or come in contact with dust, and your body, in response to the antigen, forms a bad antibody. The bad antibody joins with the antigen. Instead of solving the problem, chemicals such as histamines are given off. These chemicals are called neurotransmitters. They interfere with the normal impulses that run through your brain.

If they affect a part of your brain that controls how you feel, you may feel sad. If they affect a part of the brain that controls verbal skills then you might have trouble speaking. If they affect a part of the brain that controls coordination then you might have trouble walking, etc.[1]

Some allergic reactions may be recognized by the traditional allergist; however, many may not. Allergic reactions that show up as brain allergies and alter the way you feel or think, for instance, may or may not be accompanied by an elevated IgE level in the blood. If they are not, the traditional allergist will most likely fail to link your mental state to an allergy. In fact, since the general public and the vast majority of physicians do not associate mental problems with allergies, you would probably not go to an allergist for your fatigue or depression or for your child's hyperactivity in the first place.

However, as pointed out by Dr. Rapp, clinical ecologists recognize the role of allergies in a broad spectrum of disorders, both physical and mental. They believe that as technology advances we will someday be able to isolate the exact immune response that is causing allergic symptoms, just as we have already isolated IgE and other immunoglobulins. In the meantime, they ask, which is more important – the scientific explanation of an illness, or the attempt to treat it?

SENSITIVITY DEFINED

Because the term *allergy* came to have a narrow immunological definition, the orthodox medical establishment, especially traditional allergists, deny that what the clinical ecologists treat is, in fact, allergy. According to the orthodox view, if there is no measurable rise in IgE or other immunoglobulin, there is no allergy. To avoid squabbling over semantics, clinical ecologists developed the concept of *sensitivity*, which encompasses allergies recognized by the traditional allergist and further encompasses altered reactions to substances that do not manifest as IgE antibodies and that cannot be explained by the antigen-antibody theory. Brain "allergy," for example, is a reaction to an environmental substance; it is not readily explicable in antigen-antibody terms.

Basically the concept of *sensitivity* is synonomous with the original definition of an allergy as an "altered reaction" to a substance in a person's environment. This definition allows for medical treatment of the ever-increasing incidence of adverse reactions people are exhibiting to new and untested substances in their environment. In this book the terms *allergy* and *sensitivity* are used interchangeably, unless reference is specifically being made to the narrower, orthodox-medical definition of allergy.

THE INDIVIDUAL NATURE OF ALLERGY

"One man's meat is another man's poison," wrote Lucretius, the Roman poet and philosopher. About allergies, no truer words were ever spoken.

We saw in Case Two that Angela was sensitive to a chemical in her environment that had no noticeable effect on her husband Tony. The same phenomenon is true of food. For instance, you may be able to eat beef, but your best friend may get a migraine headache whenever she eats it. Or you may be chronically fatigued by an allergy to milk, but your son's allergy to milk may show up as hyperactivity.

Allergy is a very individual disease. By definition, it has to do with the way *you* in particular interact with your particular environment. Your allergy could have symptoms ranging from nausea to arthritis to schizophrenia.

Many people become sensitive to foods that they eat on a regular basis. Theron G. Randolph, M.D., one of the foremost clinical ecologists in this country, and Ralph Moss state in their book *An Alternative Approach to Allergies* that "any food can be abused by overeating it. If a food is eaten in any form once in three days, or more frequently, there is the chance it is being abused and may become a problem for the consumer."[2] When a food is "abused," the body incorrectly perceives the food as a foreign substance and defends against it by means of an allergic reaction.

When an individual's body cannot accept the intrusion of a factor in the environment, ecological illness occurs, often in the form of chronic disorders involving several body systems. For example, an allergy to milk may make you nauseous at first; this would be a gastrointestinal reaction. Then later you may become very fatigued, which may be due to reactions in the brain and the central nervous system.

As Timmy, and Angela discovered as a result of their doctors' extensive testing, allergies can produce symptoms so complex and varied that sufferers can be diagnosed as neurotic. Allergies can even cause behavior that may be diagnosed as psychotic. Unfortunately, many sufferers are unaware of their symptoms' underlying cause, and many physicians, including allergists, are equally in the dark because they have been trained to recognize only certain types of reactions as allergic.

The most common symptoms experienced by those sensitive to a food, chemical, or other environmental factor are:

- chronic fatigue
- headache
- insomnia
- rapid mood swings
- confusion
- depression
- anxiety
- hyperactivity
- heart palpitations
- muscle aches and joint pains
- bed-wetting
- swollen nose membranes
- hives
- shortness of breath
- diarrhea
- constipation

Clinical ecologists give particular attention to the foods a person ingests, but they also look at the whole environment, or "ecology," of the person. Clinical ecologists have found that many of today's "diseases," such as arthritis, hyperactivity in children, depression, and chronic fatigue, can be caused by an individual's sensitivity to a food or chemical in his or her environment.

DIAGNOSTIC DIFFICULTIES

Allergies are often difficult to diagnose because they can show up in any bodily organ at any time.

- James has a cerebral (brain) allergy to wheat and a gastrointestinal allergy to milk. After a breakfast of whole wheat toast and milk, James suffers immediate diarrhea due to his gastrointestinal allergy; then, several hours later, he suffers intense fatigue from his brain allergy. One meal causes two responses in two different bodily organs at two different times.

• Janet becomes either drowsy after a meal or disoriented several hours after inhaling an insect repellent, a hydrocarbon that has been shown to cause both physical and mental allergic reactions.

Such cases are difficult to diagnose. Allergic symptoms are incredibly diversified because *any* organ system can react to an allergen, and *different foods can effect different reactions in the same individual!*

Given the number and complexity of factors involved, it is no wonder that patients and physicians alike fail to see the connection between environment and allergy.

Dr. Randolph points out that these diagnostic difficulties are further compounded by what he terms "hidden addictions." He explains that many food allergies are "hidden" or "masked," not only to the patient but also to the physician. He explains how a milk sensitivity can develop, for example:

> Let us say, for instance, that you developed an allergy to milk early in life. At first this may have resulted in acute reactions such as a rash or a cough. In time, if the allergy was not recognized and controlled, the symptoms may have become more generalized and less easily detected. Since you probably went on drinking milk or eating milk products almost every day, one day's symptoms blurred into the next day's. You developed a chronic disease, such as arthritis, migraine, or depression. ...
>
> In fact you were probably abusing milk. You had become a milk junkie, a milk-o-holic. It is in the nature of this problem that a sudden loss of the craved substance can cause withdrawal symptoms. Since removal of the milk brought on a particularly bad attack of the symptoms, you unconsciously learned to keep yourself on a maintenance dose. Milk in the morning with cereal, yogurt for lunch, a glass of milk with your dinner, and, of course, a platter of cheese before retiring.[3]

Dr. Randolph refers to this type of food allergy as an addiction because the discontinuation of the given food can result in actual withdrawal symptoms, while its continued ingestion results in a temporary stimulatory effect or high.

Virtually all of the clinical ecologists stated that allergies are probably the most misdiagnosed illness in America today.[4] Allergists conservatively estimate that approximately 15 percent of the population suffers from a minimum of one allergy that is serious enough to warrant medical attention. In his book *Coping with Food Allergy*, Dr. Claude Frazier states that "from 20 to 30 million Americans, young and old, are unable to tolerate the ordinary things of this world, they react to them with illness.[5]

HOW ALLERGIES DEVELOP

THE ALLERGY-THRESHOLD CONCEPT   How do people become sensitive to foods or chemicals in their environment?

In this technological age, when literally hundreds of new chemicals are introduced into our environment each year in the form of food additives, pesticides, and cleaning solutions (to name a few), our bodies are under constant assault. Our immune systems do their best to defend us against these foreign substances. Sometimes, however, either because of the immune system's weakened condition or because of the quantity of these foreign substances (or a combination of the two), a breakdown occurs that can manifest as an allergic reaction. One explanation for this is the "allergy-threshold concept."

Dr. Rapp provides an example of this concept:

> Suppose you have a natural gas leak in your house. The furnace breaks down, and everyone is exposed to gas. Subsequent to that exposure, if you put gasoline in your car, you might get a headache or dizzy. If you walk into a kitchen with a natural gas stove, you will find that you smell gas before anyone else. Even your nose has been sensitized to the gas because your body does not want it around. ...
>
> If you have had a massive exposure to one chemical, you might find yourself sensitive to minute exposure to a wide variety of chemicals that never caused you difficulty before. For example, you put new synthetic carpets all through your house, and foam in the walls for insulation. You become sensitized to these particular chemicals. Then, when you go to church on Sunday, you might find that the smell of incense or perfume bothers you. You may find that you can't use scented soap or scented toilet paper. You may find the smell of scouring powder bothers you. You may find that there are certain stores you can no longer go in. Once you be-

come sensitized to a chemical, it is as though a switch has been flipped, and you are now sensitive to a wide variety of substances unrelated to the chemical that originally caused the problem.[6]

According to the allergy threshold concept, an individual may go over his or her threshold of tolerance because of a variety of factors both internal and external. Examples of these factors are weather, environmental pollutants, genetic predisposition, emotional stress, nutritional deficiencies, immune status, and age. These can conspire to lower the threshold, increasing the individual's susceptibility to adverse health reactions.

We are coming to realize the unfortunate truth that external pollution causes internal pollution. The barrage of chemicals introduced into our environment over the past two centuries has disrupted nature's balance. Pesticides, herbicides, and insecticides are ingested, along with the additives and preservatives that are added during the processing of foods.

In many cases the contamination of food is irreversible. For instance, chemical solvents that are used to spray fruit penetrate through to pulp and cannot be removed by washing or peeling.

It is estimated that more than 10 percent of the U.S. population has a noticeable reaction to food additives. Processed and packaged goods such as Jell-O, ice cream, sherbet, cookies, candy, and soda may contain significant amounts of food additives. Oranges, sweet potatoes, and butter may be dyed and sold without warning labels to alert the consumer. Almost all food coloring is made from synthetic dyes, among which analine and coal-tar derivatives are the most dangerous. Citrus fruits are fumigated for pest control. Commercially prepared fruits and vegetables, including those sold at salad bars, may be treated with sulfur dioxide to retard spoilage and discoloration.

For someone with allergic sensitivities to sulfur dioxide or corn products, eating out or indeed eating at all can become difficult unless extreme care is taken. Corn kernels treated with sulfur dioxide retain that chemical; it later shows up in a host of corn products, such as corn flour, cornstarch, corn syrup, corn oil, and popcorn.[7]

Most commercially raised meats and poultry are riddled with drug residues. Animals are routinely given drugs and hormones to increase their appetite, antibiotics to prevent disease, and tranquilizers before slaughter. Another common practice is to dip certain fish in an anti-biotic solution to retard spoilage. Drug-sensitive people continuously ingest drugs with their daily food consumption, provoking long- or short-term symptoms, the sources of which often go unidentified.

In addition to toxic residues in certain foods, we are subjected to the by-products of industrialization that pollute our air, water, and food supply. These chemicals, whether natural or synthetic, are foreign to the human body and cause internal pollution. Chemicals pollute the environment at a rate faster than the human body can adapt to them. We can tolerate only so much contamination before this toxic overload leads to illness.

HEREDITY Heredity may also play a decisive role in whether you suffer from allergies. If both your parents suffer from allergies, there is at least a 75 percent chance that you have inherited the condition. If one parent is allergic, you have a 50 percent chance.

A child, however, does not necessarily inherit the *same* allergic response. Joey has eczema; his mother is asthmatic. Joey's allergy is to milk; his mother's is to wheat.

With respect to allergy and heredity, Dr. Rapp says:

> You should tend to think of allergy [to explain odd behavior] if there is a lot of allergy in your family. If you have parents with hay fever or asthma, or children with hay fever or asthma, and if you have one child with behavior or personality problems, allergy could be the cause. The same milk or dust that causes asthma in one child could cause bed-wet-ting or behavioral problems in another. Any history of allergy is going to make a person more apt to have brain allergy than a person who has never heard of allergy. Parents and children often have the same allergy.[8]

Heredity may simply cause a predisposition to allergy – to any al-lergy – or it may pass a specific allergy on from parent to child. In addition, babies can develop allergies to the same foods that their mothers are allergic to, either through the placenta while they are still in the womb or through breast milk after birth. Says Dr. Rapp,

> I have known unborn babies who would hiccup or kick hard enough in the womb to bruise the mother. These mothers should think of what they ate a half hour before the baby started to act this way. If they do,

they may be able to figure out what is bothering the baby down in the uterus. One woman found that every time she ate a cannoli her baby began to kick her. The baby was having a prenatal allergic reaction and was attempting to tell the mother not to eat cannolis.

The same thing might happen after the baby is born. If a baby is totally breast-feeding and that baby becomes agitated after feeding, that mother should ask herself what she ate the previous meal. The food can come through the breast milk and make the baby sick.[9]

NUTRITIONAL DEFICIENCIES   What we eat plays an important role in whether we develop allergies. As pointed out above, continuous long-term consumption of a given food may result in an allergy to that food. It is estimated that the typical American diet consists of approximately 25 percent dairy products and an additional 25 percent wheat products in one form or another (e.g., milk, yogurt, ice cream, butter, cheese, bread, cereal, pastries, and other dough products). Consumption of these products in these proportions not only sets the stage for specific allergies to wheat and dairy but also contributes to nutritional deficiencies arising from such a restricted diet. The vitamins and minerals available from a well-balanced diet of various grains, legumes, fruits, and vegetables in the quantities necessary for proper nutrition are simply not present when almost half the foods consumed comes in two forms.

Other factors that may contribute to nutritional deficiencies include refined carbohydrates and sugars, drugs, alcohol, caffeine, cigarettes, stress, and illness. These factors weaken our immune system and inhibit its ability to function properly. The allergies recognized by orthodox allergists are by definition caused by a defective immune response to a substance in an individual's environment that that person's immune system perceives as dangerous. Although we do not yet have the technology to detect the immune response to fatigue, tension, and migraines that manifests in the subtler forms of allergy recognized by clinical ecologists, most clinical ecologists believe that the subtler forms of allergy are in fact caused by some type of immune response. If this is the case, proper nutrition becomes doubly important in preventing allergies since it also serves to ensure a strong, healthy immune system.

THREE-WAY ATTACK

Allergic substances can enter our bodies in three ways. *Ingestants* enter through the digestive system via foods, beverages, and drugs. *Inhalants* enter through the respiratory system via pollens, molds, dust, animal dander, or chemicals. And still other substances enter through the skin via poison ivy, insect bites, direct contact with chemicals in household cleaners, perfumes, suntan lotion, shaving cream, cosmetics, and the like.

Repeated exposure to these allergens starts the process of sensitization in those who are susceptible. It can lead to a breakdown in healthy physical and mental functioning. With foods this sensitization occurs in response to those eaten most frequently. For the general population foods most likely to cause trouble are milk, wheat, corn, sugar, beef, eggs, citrus fruits, potatoes, yeast, and tomatoes.

THREE TYPES OF ALLERGIC RESPONSE

FIXED ALLERGIC RESPONSES *Fixed* allergies cause a reaction every time the offending food is consumed. For example, if you have a fixed allergy to strawberries, a reaction occurs whenever you eat strawberries, no matter how long you've abstained from them or how few you've eaten. Whether you bite into a fresh strawberry or eat strawberry jam, your face breaks out in hives. If you were unaware of what causes your hives, your physician would detect the allergen through testing or a comprehensive case history.

CYCLIC ALLERGIC RESPONSES *Cyclic* allergies, unlike fixed allergies, do not appear each and every time you eat a food, but rather they depend upon the frequency of your consumption of the food. Effects of cyclic allergies are cumulative. If you eat a food to which you have a cyclic allergy daily, the food builds up in your system and is never fully eliminated. In that case one day's symptoms blur into the next day's, resulting in symptoms such as chronic fatigue or depression. It is just such chronic symptoms that traditional allergists may fail to identify as allergies and that the medical community is more apt to treat as a psychological or psychiatric problem. Clinical ecologists, however, recognize the role that foods and environmental allergens play in chronic fatigue, mood changes, and behavior patterns.

If you were to visit a clinical ecologist for these types of symptoms, you would probably first be put on an *elimination diet* to rid your body of any residue of the food. Through *provocative testing* the clinical ecologist would (hopefully) discover the substance to which you were allergic, then relieve your symptoms by finding the *neutralizing dose* of that substance.

Unless you were intolerably allergic to the substance, you would then be put on a *four-day rotational diet*, in which you could still consume that food but no more often than once every four days.

ADDICTIVE-ALLERGIC RESPONSES AND THE TENSION FATIGUE SYNDROME   The *addictive-allergic* response is the type of allergy (described by Dr. Randolph above) that often remains hidden because the patient actively craves the allergenic food, feels better for a while after having eaten it, and then suffers withdrawal symptoms as the amount of that allergen in the body decreases. This type of physical response is similar for alcohol, sugar, nicotine, caffeine, and other types of addictive agents. In effect, when your body craves any substance, you may be developing an addiction to that substance.

The addictive-allergic response is often accompanied by what is commonly referred to as the *tension-fatigue syndrome*.

Here's an example of how the addictive-allergic response and the tension-fatigue syndrome show up in a child. Ten-year-old Bobby loves junk food. His mother tries to feed him wholesome food, but he refuses to eat it and wants only what he sees advertised on television: packaged cereals, soda pop, candy, and the like. He is a source of constant worry for his mother. At one moment Bobby is energetic – too energetic. He can't sit still, he knocks things over, he is into everything, he causes trouble at school, and at times he even appears to have spasmodic muscular movements. At the next moment Bobby is depressed, lethargic, almost catatonic, and unwilling to do anything at all.

After Bobby visits a clinical ecologist, it is determined that Bobby is reacting to the large amounts of food additives in his diet. Much to his dismay – and to his mother's delight – the doctor puts Bobby on a diet that is substantially free of these food additives. As long as Bobby stays on the diet he is "normal." The moment he resumes his old eating patterns his behavioral problems flare up again.

In the tension-fatigue syndrome, an allergic response begins as a stimulation, causing tension and often hyperactivity. Then as the effects of the food wear off, extreme fatigue and exhaustion are experienced.

Another example, given by Dr. Randolph, shows how tension-fatigue caused by an addictive allergy can affect us:

> Charles Henderson, a prominent businessman, came to see me because he was troubled by mental exhaustion, mental confusion, and fatigue. He was a top executive of a large company who dictated to a battery of secretaries from morning to night. One of his secretaries pointed out to him that he did not give understandable dictation during the late afternoon. This was hard for her, because Henderson usually scolded her the next day for not accurately reproducing his previous day's dictation.
>
> In desperation, the secretary suggested that Henderson relax with the office staff in the afternoon and have a snack. Once he did so she was able to comprehend his words and directions somewhat better. For this man, a snack meant only one thing: eggs. In fact, he had eggs for breakfast, egg salad for lunch, and some dessert containing eggs at dinner almost every day. His secretary literally "egged him on" to have eggs at break time, as well.
>
> When I finished taking the man's history, I told him, "Mr. Henderson, I think you are allergic to eggs."
>
> He jumped from his chair and said, "Doctor, you obviously didn't understand what I just told you! Let me repeat it: Eggs are the one food I *know* agrees with me. Now you tell me I may be allergic to them. That doesn't make any sense to me at all." He was clearly on the point of walking out of the office. He knew what he was allergic to and what he wasn't.
>
> This episode took place in the late 1940s. I had just finished a rather intensive study of drug addiction and had privately reached the conclusion that food allergy and drug addiction were aspects of the same problem. I decided to explain the problem to Henderson in terms of addiction. I explained that he seemed to have a three-hour "high" from eggs, after which he started to come down, with attendant symptoms of confusion and fatigue. He had to eat eggs every three hours or so in order to remain "high."

This made some sense to him, and he agreed to take a test to prove its validity. Since it takes between two and three days to clear any particular meal from the intestines, Henderson ate no eggs, or product containing eggs, during the next few days. He suffered from withdrawal symptoms, and was so weak that he could not get out of bed to go to work.

He began to feel better after the eggs were entirely out of his system. Then he came back to my office, where he was fed eggs in a testing room. Within less than an hour, he had returned these eggs, through violent projectile vomiting, halfway across the room. He was terribly embarrassed, but amazed to see that his "favorite" food really did not agree with him at all.

By staying off eggs for six months or so he was able to break his addiction to them. After that, he was able to reintroduce eggs into his diet, but only once every four days, in order to prevent the addiction from re-forming. By controlling this and other food allergies, he was able to restore his ability to think and dictate clearly.[10]

ALLERGIES AND CHILDREN

As pointed out above by Dr. Rapp, food allergies can commence as early as the prenatal months. Prenatal allergies can cause babies to kick and punch in their mothers' womb. As infants they may drool excessively or require frequent formula change due to chronic colic. As children they may be hyperactive, and if they suffer from brain allergies, they often have dark circles under their eyes. Chronic ear complications often occur before the age of one and persist on into the toddler years. As tots, they are commonly plagued by temper tantrums, leg aches, and crying spells. Many of these children do not laugh or smile until they are two years old.

By the age of six they often experience gastrointestinal problems such as bloating, gas, diarrhea, and constipation. Respiratory difficulties, headaches, and fatigue are also common. During the teen years they may suffer from marked mood swings. Adulthood symptoms may involve a combination of those previously experienced, such as gastrointestinal or respiratory difficulties; or, as is often the case, a stimulatory response such as childhood hyperactivity may turn into withdrawal symptoms, insomnia, or depression.[11]

Dr. Rapp gives examples of how brain allergies can affect a child's behavior:

I saw an eighteen-year-old girl who, according to her mother, punched her way out of the uterus. Behaviorally, she was one problem after another. She had classical nose and chest allergies. She noticed that she always became tired and depressed when she visited one particular friend's house. She told us that in that house she always smelled natural gas. The house had a gas stove and gas heat. Without her knowing what we were testing for, we tested her for natural gas. We bubbled natural gas through saline and placed a drop of this beneath her tongue. She developed the same behavioral abnormalities that she had exhibited at her friend's house. I remember this girl was so sensitive to chemicals that once, after using fingernail polish, she sat in the middle of the street trying to get hit by a car. Once, with her boyfriend, she was exposed to gasoline fumes and did something to try and kill herself.

In another case one boy, three years old, fussed and cried when visiting Grandma. He became an impossible youngster. Grandma's house smelled of natural gas, and she used natural gas heat. We tested the boy for natural gas, again bubbling the gas through a saline solution and placing a drop of this beneath the boy's tongue. Soon he started to whine and cry.[12]

ADDRESSING ALL NEGATIVE FACTORS

For both you and your doctor, the proper treatment of your allergies may require a significant amount of time and dedication. As the name implies, clinical ecology is concerned with your whole environment and the way you interact with it. Elimination of the offending food may not be enough to obtain optimal health unless the rest of your environment and lifestyle is also healthy.

It may not be possible to eliminate all the pollutants and stress factors from your twentieth-century life, but it is possible to mitigate the effects these factors may have on your allergies in particular, and on your health in general. Proper diet, stress reduction, and adequate exercise all can build a healthy immune system and increase your resistance to allergies.

Proper food combining is also important. Although you may tolerate a specific food when you eat it alone, it may provoke or aggravate an allergic response when combined with other foods. For instance, you may be allergic to dairy products; they may give you mild headaches. But you could find that when you eat dairy products with wheat – as in a grilled cheese sandwich – you get not a mild headache but a splitting migraine. Or you may find that you can eat beef alone, but when you eat hamburgers – beef plus wheat – your arthritis flares up.

Sometimes allergic reactions occur or are aggravated by the length of time the allergen is in your system. Digestive problems or constipation may also add to your allergies. Faulty digestion can also allow improperly digested molecules of food into your bloodstream; the immune system then mistakes them for foreign substances. This, too, can cause allergies.

The quality and quantity of a food allergen can also be a factor. Coffee, tobacco, and alcohol, for example, are highly potent allergens for most people. Used over prolonged periods of time, especially in large amounts, they can cause very severe reactions. Dairy products, wheat, and beef, which constitute the major part of most Americans' diets day in and day out, are also particularly potent allergens when consumed in the large quantities in which most people consume them.

Once one allergy has set in, it often paves the way for other allergies. One clinical study has shown that the average person suffering from hay fever is also allergic to five foods. Those with allergic rhinitis (swelling of the nasal membranes) had, on the average, seven allergies, and those with asthma had ten. This study indicates that food sensitivities are closely related to other forms of allergy and often precipitate symptoms similar to those caused by allergens.

BREAKDOWN

Many diseases, if carefully analyzed, can be traced to the persistent, long-term use of a substance that is unhealthy either in itself or when consumed over long periods of time. Lung cancer can be traced to cigarettes; some experts claim prostate cancer can be traced to meat products. These are but two examples. Often the adverse effects of these substances initially show up as a minor symptom or illness. It is only after these symptoms are ignored or masked by drugs over time that a serious illness or breakdown occurs, caused by the body's inability to fight off the noxious effects of the substance.

Repeated or prolonged weakening of the body by recurrent allergic reactions has the same breakdown effect. This breakdown may affect one or more parts of the body. It is usually severe enough to cause a person to consult a physician. However, doctor and patient are both usually unaware of the history of and underlying factors behind the symptom. Both falsely assume that the symptom signifies the *beginning* of an illness rather than seeing that it is a distress signal of a disorder initiated years before by an allergy.

I would argue that in some cases arthritis is caused by a breakdown due to food allergies; it is often diagnosed by orthodox medicine, however, as a "primary" disease rather than as a result of long-term allergic reactions.

Breakdown may be preceded by a long period of sensitivity. Yet the connection between prior and present symptoms is often ignored by traditional practitioners. If, for instance, your allergic response takes the form of eczema, palpitations, and abdominal pains, you may seek the advice of a dermatologist, a cardiologist, and an internist. Each specialist then will treat each symptom independently of the others, when in fact all complaints may be caused by sensitivity to one or more environmental factors.

TREATMENT

THE ELIMINATION DIET   Many food allergies are of the cyclic and allergic-addictive nature, in which an allergenic food is tolerated; you don't break out in a rash or start sneezing or coughing immediately upon eating it. So it is important to cleanse the body of all residues of the allergenic food that have built up in your body over the years. This is done both to relieve your symptoms and to begin the diagnostic process of determining exactly which substances are at the root of your allergy.

This cleansing process is the *elimination diet*. It is used by both traditional allergists and clinical ecologists in the process of determining food allergies. There is substantial agreement between the two types of allergists about the importance of the elimination diet in diagnosing food allergies and about how the diet is utilized, although clinical ecologists may be more rigorous about the elimination of substances and about the duration of the diet. The elimination diet is also used to diagnose fixed allergies when the source of the allergy is undetermined.

The elimination diet, as recommended by clinical ecologists, usually lasts one week. During this week the most common allergenic foods, such as wheat, dairy, corn, and beef *in all forms*, are eliminated from your diet, in addition to any foods that your particular case history reveal as being troublesome to you. If you have particularly severe symptoms, you may even be requested to go on a water fast in order to completely cleanse your system.

PROVOCATIVE TESTING AND NEUTRALIZING DOSE   Once you have finished your elimination diet, the next phase in the diagnosis of your allergies is *provocative testing.* It works like this. You and your doctor suspect that you have an allergy to wheat. You have been on an elimination diet to cleanse your body of wheat residue. Your doctor then tests you with an extract of wheat in a certain dilution, either by placing a drop of it under your tongue or by injecting it into the skin. Your responses are measured. If you are in fact allergic, you will manifest the symptoms of which you previously complained. Your doctor monitors changes in your pulse, lung and nasal functions, blood pressure, heart rate, and the like. Once this provocative testing determines that you are allergic to wheat, your doctor will continue to test you with progressively weaker dilutions of the wheat extract until he or she arrives at the exact dilution that neutralizes your symptoms. This dilution is called the *neutralizing dose.* It has been shown to relieve both IgE- and non-IgE-mediated allergies more rapidly and effectively than drug therapy.[13]

The neutralizing dose is especially useful in cases where avoidance of an allergen is difficult or impossible, or where multiple food allergies are present.

There is as yet no scientific explanation of how and why the neutralizing dose of an allergen relieves the symptoms caused by the same allergen. It is thought to work in the same way that the *infinitesimal dose* works in homeopathic remedies; this unfortunately is also unexplainable scientifically. Nevertheless, it has been shown to work clinically, often with the same efficacy as drugs and without the harmful side effects.

The provocative testing/neutralizing dose method of treatment can often detect allergies that would be undetectable by normal or traditional testing methods. It then provides a safe, nontoxic treatment for the allergy. This is especially important in cases of schizophrenia, manic depression, and other psychiatric disorders that are often treated with drugs whose toxic side effects are more severe than the diseases they are meant to treat.

FOUR-DAY ROTATIONAL DIET   Once the source of your allergy has been determined, your doctor will prescribe a four-day rotational diet for you. In most cases you will be asked to eliminate the offending food altogether, at least at first. Other foods will then be rotated on a four-day basis so that you do not develop any new allergies. Later, your doctor may allow you to reintroduce the offending food back into your diet, provided that you eat it no more than once every four days.

The neutralizing dose and the four-day rotational diet are both treatment aspects of clinical ecology. But each addresses a different type of allergic reaction. The neutralizing dose is used primarily when you cannot tolerate a food at all without a severe reaction, or when it may be impossible for you to avoid it. For example, you may have respiratory problems every time you eat mustard, sometimes almost to the point of suffocation. You go to a friend's house for dinner; unaware of your allergy, the friend uses mustard in the salad dressing. After eating the salad you have a severe attack. The neutralizing dose may be used to subdue that symptom.

The four-day rotational diet, on the other hand, is used if your allergy to a food allows you to eat the food occasionally but makes you depressed and apathetic if it is eaten regularly.

In certain cases the neutralization dosage may be used in conjunction with the four-day rotational diet. Children who are allergic to wheat and milk, for example, may be able to eat birthday cake and ice cream without too much trouble if they use the neutralizing dose; or people who are allergic to oats may be able to have oatmeal for breakfast, provided they do so no more than once every four days.

A CONTROLLED ENVIRONMENT   Elimination and four-day rotational diets and neutralization therapy help in the diagnosis and treatment of ecological disorders. However, in the clinical experience of some physicians, such tests work best under environmentally controlled hospital conditions, especially in advanced cases, where the patient has multiple symptoms and multiple offending allergens. Such people need to clear their systems of all allergens for four to seven days before testing can begin. This assures greater accuracy. In a controlled hospital setting, patients fast on distilled water for at least three days before the testing procedures begin. This is a small sacrifice for the relief they experience once the source of their symptoms is identified.

CORRECTING IMBALANCES   Another part of the comprehensive treatment of environmental allergies is the **correction of vitamin, mineral, and enzyme imbalances.** Some doctors have had success with vitamin C, vitamin B_6, and niacin.

A patient's diet may also be supplemented by betaine hydrochloride and digestive enzymes to facilitate digestion, for underlying many food allergies is an impaired digestive system. For proper digestion, it is imperative that sufficient hydrochloric acid be secreted into the stomach, along with pancreatic enzymes. These substances break down the large protein molecules into small molecules so that they are easier to absorb and utilize.

When there is too little secretion of the digestive juices and enzymes, large protein molecules go directly into the bloodstream. The immune system then reacts to these large molecules as if they were foreign invaders, causing an allergic response.

To alleviate these allergies, it is vital to restore the digestive system to optimal function. Balancing the digestive enzymes is, therefore, a key issue.

DRUGS ARE NOT THE ANSWER   One of the major differences between clinical ecologists and the orthodox medical community is their attitude toward drugs. Although clinical ecologists acknowledge the efficacy of drugs and the appropriateness of their prescription in certain cases, they consider drugs a treatment of last resort. Clinical ecologists are qualified medical doctors and in many cases are board-certified specialists. They are conscious of the Hippocratic oath, which dictates, "First, do no harm." Drugs may be effective in allaying certain symptoms, and they may also be curative, as are some antibiotics.

But most drugs have many toxic side effects. Some of the most toxic drugs are those used in the treatment of psychiatric disorders such as Thorazine, Stelazine, and Haldol. Not only do these drugs produce allergic skin reactions, hepatitis, brain damage, and liver destruction in some patients; they are also attributable to tardive dyskinesia, a central nervous system disorder. This disorder is characterized by spasmodic muscle movements such as grimacing, sticking one's tongue out, and blinking. Some physicians believe these movements are caused by brain damage as a result of prolonged use of toxic drugs. Tardive dyskinesia is incurable, and it does not go away when drug intake is discontinued. Its existence raises the question of which is more pernicious: the mental disorder or its treatment.

Because the side effects of these "antipsychotic" drugs are severe, alternatives are worth investigating, such as the approach of clinical ecologists. They may be able to treat mental diseases simply by eliminating an allergenic food from the diet or with a nontoxic neutralization dosage of that food.

Another disadvantage of using drugs as a primary mode of therapy that clinical ecologists note is that most drugs treat only the symptoms and not the cause of a disease. Over twenty-five hundred years ago Hippocrates advised, "Let thy food be thy medicine and thy medicine be thy food. Leave your drugs in the chemist's pot if you can heal the patient with food."

Roger J. Williams, Ph.D., professor of nutritional science at the Clayton Biochemical Institute of the University of Texas at Austin, is a pioneer in the field of nutrition. He echoes Hippocrates in saying:

> Drugs are wholly unlike nature's weapons. They tend to mask the difficulty not eliminate it. They contaminate the internal environment, create dependence on the part of the patient, and often complicate the physician's job by erasing valuable clues as to the real source of the trouble.[15]

Patients and the general public have begun to respond with doubt and mistrust when drugs or psychiatric evaluations are prescribed as answers to every ill. And justifiably so: in many cases doctors overmedicate their patients, resulting in a staggering incidence of physician-induced illness. In one year alone Americans took over 1.5 million pounds of tranquilizers, more than 800,000 pounds of barbiturates, and 4 million pounds of penicillin.[16]

SKEPTICISM IN THE MEDICAL PROFESSION   Dr. Rapp explains that orthodox doctors are still very skeptical of clinical ecology. She says that this is because "we cannot explain to everyone's satisfaction, including our own, why a dilution of milk [a neutralization dosage] would enable somebody to drink milk without vomiting, without getting hyperactive. But that's how it works. It doesn't mean that our observations aren't valid; it means that we just aren't smart enough right now to explain why it works."[17]

Clearly, more research is needed to understand what occurs on the cellular level. Meanwhile, more and more people are becoming dissatisfied with traditional medical approaches and are seeking answers from clinical ecology that go beyond the boundaries of traditional health care. Sadly, however, clinical ecology has been slow to gain respect and recognition from the mainstream medical community, despite its enthusiastic reception by the public and its documented successes.

AN ALLERGY CHECKLIST

The following checklist shows symptoms that may indicate the presence of an allergy or allergies. If a clinical ecologist suspects a patient is suffering from allergies, he or she may begin by inquiring about these symptoms. As you read down the list, notice whether any of the symptoms apply to you. If so, you may wish to consult a qualified health practitioner for diagnosis and treatment.

SYMPTOMS IN INFANCY AND CHILDHOOD

Colic as an infant
Difficulty gaining weight
Skin rashes
Frequent illnesses
Difficulty sleeping
Traditionally recognized
    allergic reactions
    (asthma, hives, etc.)
Earaches or fluid in the ears
Runny or stuffy nose
Coughing or wheezing
Muscle aches
"Growing pains"
Constipation
Diarrhea
Dark circles under eyes
Bags or puffiness under
    eyes

Swollen glands
Sore throat
Stomachaches
Headaches
Bed-wetting (after age three)

Glassy eyes after eating
Pale face
Behavioral problems
Learning disabilities
Short attention span
Hyperactivity

SYMPTOMS IN ADULTHOOD

Physical Symptoms

Digestive problems: gas,
  bloating, belching
Abdominal distension
Stomachaches
Constipation or diarrhea
Rectal itching
Stuffy or runny nose
Sinus problems
Headaches
Muscle aches
Loss of physical coordination
Dark circles, bags or
  puffiness under eyes

Watery eyes
"Sand" in eyes
Sore throat
Phlegm in throat
Coughing or wheezing
Sneezing
Rapid heartbeat after eating
Heart palpitations after
  eating
Rapid pulse after eating
Joint pain
Swollen joints
Difficulty urinating, water
  retention
Red earlobes after eating

Emotional Symptoms

Fatigue
Drowsiness
Insomnia
Irritability
Mood Swings
Depression
Crying
Anxiety

Paranoia
Schizophrenic behavior
Tendency to get angry easily
Nervousness
Loss of memory
Difficulty concentrating

Symptoms Related to Eating

Compulsive eating
Binging

Certain foods improve mood
Feeling better or worse

Craving specific foods, such
 as bread, tomatoes, ice
 cream
Feeling strong aversion to
 certain foods

after eating
Addiction to alcohol or drugs

Family History

One or both parents with
 traditional allergies

Family members who
 experience any of the
 above symptoms

CHAPTER TWO

Allergies and Mental Health

CASE ONE Sixteen-year-old Peter was arrested for punching his employer and assigned to juvenile probation. His medical history was investigated, and it revealed previous erratic behavior. He was sometimes normal, and sometimes disobedient, irate, and violent. Peter also had a history of seizures that led to blackouts. A high level of aluminum in Peter's blood had been thought to cause the seizures, so his aluminum level was being controlled by drugs.

Peter's probation counselor wisely sent the boy to a clinical ecologist, who put Peter on an elimination diet. Peter revealed during an interview that he had been drinking up to eight glasses of milk a day for as long as he could remember. During the second week of the diet, when dairy products were eliminated, Peter's seizures halted. Later reintroduction of dairy products caused several seizures in one day.

Prognosis: Observance of a dairy-free diet should greatly reduce the incidence of Peter's seizures and antisocial behavior.

CASE TWO Mary, age five, had suffered from typical allergies like hay fever, asthma, and skin rashes since she was three. She had dark circles and puffiness under her eyes. Behaviorally, she was an impossible child. Her parents complained that she was hyperactive, irritable, "into everything," and couldn't sit still; she made car travel a virtual impossibility. At school she quarreled with the other children, had no friends, and was constantly being disciplined by her teacher for disrupting the class. She had learning problems. Mary also com-

••29••

plained of headaches and stomachaches and had frequent diarrhea.

Her parents had taken her to her pediatrician numerous times. The doctor said Mary was hyperactive and after doing tests on her, learning disabled. The doctor prescribed Ritalin, an appetite suppressant. For reasons not yet understood, Ritalin often has a quieting effect on hyperactive children. The pediatrician then said that that was all he could do.

The Ritalin did quiet Mary for a while. She could sit still longer and her learning improved somewhat, but her allergies continued, as did the stomachaches and headaches, and she was often still moody and irritable. After a couple of months, though, the quieting effect of the Ritalin became inconsistent. Mary's mother began to worry about the wisdom and long-term effects of giving her five-year-old daughter an appetite suppressant during her formative years.

Taking a suggestion from a friend, Mary's mother brought her to a clinical ecologist, who put Mary on a two-week elimination diet. At the end of the two weeks Mary's mother found that Mary's disposition and attitude had markedly improved, she had begun to play normally at school, and she was calmer and more affectionate.

Testing by the clinical ecologist revealed that Mary became hyperactive and irritable in response to milk; that corn caused her to have diarrhea and stomachaches; and that chocolate, peanuts, and strawberries caused hyperactivity and headaches. Food allergies were found to be responsible for the dark circles and puffiness under Mary's eyes, for her learning disabilities and antisocial behavior, for her hyperactivity, and even for changes in her voice and in drawings she made. Mary's improvement was so dramatic that after a couple of weeks on a four-day rotational diet, Mary's teacher called to ask what drug Mary was taking.

CASE THREE   Dr. Brown, a small-town pediatrician, thought he was losing his mind. He was experiencing strange episodes during which he had visual hallucinations and seemingly lost the ability to read. Each episode, which was accompanied by severe diarrhea, lasted four days and then subsided. Dr. Brown was diagnosed and medicated as a schizophrenic.

Then Dr. Brown noticed that his hallucination spells consistently followed his eating boiled chicken. As soon as he removed boiled chicken from his diet, the spells stopped and did not recur.

The common theme of these three cases is that food sensitivities play a role in the way we think, act, and behave. That allergies and sensitivities play such a role in mental health is not readily accepted by the orthodox medical establishment. More often than not, people with marked behavioral problems are referred to psychiatrists – or in the case of children, to pediatricians – where their dietary habits are rarely studied. Instead, child and adult alike may simply be labeled according to their behavior – "schizophrenic," "hyperactive," "learning disabled," "manic depressive," and so on – or they may be given drugs to suppress their symptoms. But rarely is the allergenic cause of their disease found and eliminated.

Numerous types of mental disorders have been demonstrated to result from brain malfunctions due to food and chemical allergies. Clinical ecologists have found that symptoms of schizophrenia, depression, headache, hyperactivity and even psychosis can be induced by the introduction of certain foods or chemicals and that they can be shut off by eliminating these substances from the allergic person's environment or by administering a neutralization dosage.

Based on his own clinical observations, Dr. Theron Randolph estimates that between 60 and 70 percent of all symptoms that are diagnosed as psychosomatic are actually caused by environmental allergies. Dr. Randolph gives an example of one of his earliest cases of this:

> It was first brought home to me that allergic reactions to foods or beverages can either mimic or be a cause and a factor in emotional disturbances when I encountered a woman who drank forty cups of coffee a day, each cup sweetened with two teaspoons of beet sugar. She claimed to keep well on this regimen. As long as she drank coffee with beet sugar every half hour, she claimed to be just fine.
>
> She turned out to be violently sensitive to beets and to beet sugar and at least moderately sensitive to coffee. When these foods were removed from her diet, her depression – which had been gradually increasing in severity – subsided, and she only became depressed when she ate one of the foods she was reacting to intermittently. She could then make herself better by eating those foods every day. This is because a stimulatory response was followed a few hours later by depression unless the supply was replenished.

How was she diagnosed? Well, I took this woman who was suffering from severe depression every day, and I put her in the hospital. I told her to avoid the foods that she ate every day. She was worse for a while because of her withdrawal symptoms, and then she felt better. At the end of five days she was well. She did not complain anymore about depression, which had been plaguing her for several months.

She was in her room one evening about six o'clock eating her evening meal. Her vegetable as beets. Cane sugar was not allowed on her diet, but beet sugar was, as were beets. Since going on the diet she had not had any beets or beet sugar – until this meal. About two hours later I got a frantic call that my patient was psychotic. They wanted to know what they could do with her. Could they send her to the psychiatric floor?

I realized that this was the first material of beet origin this patient had eaten in the past five or six days. I knew this was probably an acute reaction to beets because this was the way in which we identified food allergies. We suspect a food because of its frequency in the diet, we remove the frequently eaten food from the diet completely for five or six days, and then we reintroduce the food, looking for an acute reaction.

Each time we fed this woman beets or beet sugar, she became hyperactive. This was followed by a period of depression. The depression lasted for two and a half days. We made a motion picture of this case, and I have seen thousands of similar cases.

I followed the history of this woman for many years after she was diagnosed. She was married and took a honeymoon in Hawaii. This location was selected because – allegedly – there was no beet sugar there, since it was a state that raised cane sugar. She had two reactions in Hawaii and they were traced to food that had been shipped from California canned with beet sugar.

Occasional exposure to a food allergen to which one is extremely susceptable, as in this case, will induce an acute episode of depression.[1]

William H. Philpott, M.D., a psychiatrist and a leading clinical ecologist who practices in St. Petersburg, Florida, states that out of 250 consecutive, unselected, emotionally disturbed patients treated in his practice, the majority exhibited symptoms typical of their mental illness upon exposure to commonly consumed foods and frequently encountered chemicals. Dr. Philpott calculated that 92 percent of the schizophrenic patients showed schizophrenic symptoms when exposed to certain foods or chemicals; 64 percent showed symptoms upon exposure to wheat; 51 percent to corn; 51 percent to milk; 75 percent to tobacco (of which 10 percent were psychotic); and 30 percent to petrochemicals.[2]

Dr. Philpott gives the following examples in his book *Brain Allergies* that illustrate the link between food and chemical sensitivities and mental health. These examples also show how this link is clinically established: introducing the allergen turns the symptom on, and withdrawing it turns the symptom off.

Henry, seventeen years old, had been mentally ill for three years. Prior use of tranquilizers, psychotherapy and electric shock did not succeed in helping him appreciably. He believed that people were out to kill him, and he often had to be placed under restraint because of his attacks on innocent children and adults. He was placed on a fast from all foods and given spring water only. He remained mentally ill until the fourth day, at which time his symptoms cleared; he was released from his restraints. He telephoned his parents, saying, "I love you. Please come and see me." On the fifth day of the fast he was fed a meal of wheat only. Within an hour, he began to feel strange and unreal; within an hour and a half, he thought people were going to kill him. He telephoned his parents again, saying, "I hate you. You caused my illness. I don't want to ever see you again." Further testing confirmed the fact that when specific foods were withheld, his symptoms cleared, and when given wheat again the same paranoid reaction occurred consistently.

Karl had been under treatment for paranoid schizophrenia; tranquilizers had been used with only partial success. Periodically, he thought he was Jesus Christ and that his father was God. ...

The morning of his first day in the hospital he exhibited his usual symptoms; however, he also complained of smelling gas. Based on my psychiatric training, I reasoned that this was another of Karl's delusions. I had seen many schizophrenics who said they smelled various things; I always assumed their ideas to be delusions. But by now, my clinical-ecological experience had made me question the validity of my medical training. I began to look for a source of gas. ...

It turned out that across from his room was a dumbwaiter going to the kitchen below. Around the corner from his room was a stairway leading to the kitchen. I opened the door to the stairway, and to my surprise, I, too, smelled gas. They had just cooked breakfast on a gas range below. ...

I placed him in another room which was free from any gases or other pollutants. He was also put on a fast, drinking spring water only. Each day I asked him about his symptoms. On the morning of the fourth day his symptoms were gone. I took him to our allergy-test room and, without telling him the substance I was using, placed drops of auto-exhaust-fume extract under his tongue for quick absorption into his system. In about two minutes or so he announced to me that he was Jesus Christ. I gave him 100 per cent oxygen to breathe for five minutes. When this did not help, I added a small amount of CO_2 to the oxygen; CO_2 improves the body's use of oxygen. After about two minutes of breathing oxygen and carbon dioxide, he announced that he was not Jesus Christ.

I had turned off his delusion by arranging for the avoidance of contact with petroleum products; then, when he was symptom-free, I exposed him to exhaust-fume extract which induced the symptoms within minutes. I again turned the delusion off, this time through the detoxifying effect of oxygen and carbon dioxide. The fundamental cause of the psychotic delusion was no longer a mystery.

His history revealed that three years before, while driving a propane-fueled fork truck in an apple warehouse cooler, he was overcome by the fumes from the truck, fell to the floor, and was revived by emergency oxygen. It was after this that he developed his psychosis, and these attacks had always coincided with his driving the fork truck in the apple cooler. He also reacted to several foods, but only gas fumes made him delusional. It was significant that, on one occasion when he waxed his crew-cut hair, he literally went crazy. People who are very sensitive to petrochemical hydrocarbons have to avoid items coming from petroleum sources: candles, waxes, sprays, fresheners, perfumes, certified food coloring, exhaust fumes, whitened cane sugar and anything else derived from or contaminated by petrochemical hydrocarbons.[3]

Dr. Doris Rapp gives an example of how behavioral problems in a child were found to be caused by an environmental sensitivity:

I had a nine-year-old boy who becomes very vulgar when he eats certain foods or is checked for molds. His mother found that when he went to a particular school, he tended to be vulgar in that school. We went to the school with an air pump, collected samples, and then bubbled this air through a saline solution. We took that youngster, who was sensible and normal at the time, and we made him vulgar by placing a drop of his school air allergy extract under his tongue. He became vulgar with both his speech and actions. We made him jump on the furniture and scribble on walls. He threaded to pee up his mother's leg and do very strange things. When we gave him the correct dilution [the neutralization dosage] of the school air allergy extract, he came right back to normal.[4]

Some children who are hyperactive due to allergies experience a slump in energy and even extreme fatigue after a period of hyperactivity. This parallels the tension-fatigue syndrome described in Chapter 1, in which a period of overstimulation or tension or "hyperactivity" is followed by a period of fatigue or exhaustion. Some children become so exhausted that they have to be carried home from school.

Allergies can affect our brains as much as they can affect other parts of our bodies. The brain is made up of living cells that originated from the same fertilized egg as all the other cells in our body, and hence it is just as susceptible to allergy. Brain allergies or *altered reactions* within the brain can be responsible for virtually all types of mental dysfunction, ranging from fatigue, blurred vision, and headaches to criminal behavior, schizophrenia, and psychosis. Recognition of the fact that allergies are at the root of many mental disorders could become one of our greatest medical advances.

It is estimated that nearly 1 percent of the U.S. population are patients in psychiatric hospitals in any given year and that around 10 percent will be mental patients at some time in their lives.[5] These figures do not even include the millions of patients in prisons and youth detention centers, as well as out-patients treated with antipsychotic drugs.

In traditional psychiatric practice (aside from psychotherapy) antipsychotic drugs are the primary mode of treatment for mental disorders, either alone or in conjunction with electroconvulsive therapy (and not so long ago, lobotomy). These drugs are very powerful and have extreme side effects. When chlorpromazine, the generic name for Thorazine, first appeared on the market in the early 1950s, it was described by psychiatrists as the equivalent of a "functional lobotomy."[6] Many physicians believe that the lobotomy effect is due to severe brain damage caused by the drugs. Dr. Philpott cites a study that showed a 20 percent loss of brain cells in the corpus striatum of rats injected with phenothiazine, a chemical name for Thorazine.[7]

Thorazine and other antipsychotic drugs and tranquilizers, such as Stelazine and Haldol, have other undesirable side effects, such as hepatitis, bone marrow allergies, liver damage, "silent coronary death," tardive dyskinesia, and Parkinson's disease. Dr. Philpott gives some examples:

> Peter, a 45-year-old, took Thorazine for five years. One year after taking it he had a mask-like face and walked stiffly. He was given an anti-Parkinson's medication but kept on the Thorazine because his psychotic symptoms recurred if he stopped it. Today Peter suffers from tremors and convulsions. He is diagnosed as having permanent Parkinson's disease and

these symptoms do not go away even when the Thorazine is removed.

Sally was twenty-five when she began to take the tranquilizer Haldol. Three years later she developed tardive dyskinesia. Her head jerks from side to side and her tongue moves in and out of her mouth continuously. She has odd muscle spasms in her face which resemble grimaces.[8]

The Head of the U.S. Senate Select Committee on Nutrition and Human Needs in 1977, Senator George McGovern expressed his concern at the failure and neglect of orthodox medicine to alleviate many of America's mental health problems. He stated:

Achieving recognition of the relationship between nutrition and [mental] health is still very much a struggle. Established scientific thinking remains weighted against those who are striving to understand the complex links between the food we consume and how we think and behave as individuals. For example, the newly appointed Mental Health Commission has no member with experience in this vital area. I find this oversight both surprising and distressing. ... If further research is undertaken along a nutritional line, we could find that a significant number of mental health problems could be cured or prevented by better nutrition.[9]

In many cases an environmental approach to mental illness enables doctors to get at the root cause of a disease and to actually heal the illness without the harmful side effects of drugs. We have seen in many of the examples above that simply the elimination of certain foods can bring a mentally disturbed patient back to normal.

This is not to say that all mental disorders have allergy as a root cause. Another branch of nutrition-based medicine, orthomolecular medicine, has found that some psychiatric conditions are caused by vitamin deficiencies and can be effectively treated by megadoses of the deficient nutrient. Other instances of mental disorder may have a purely psychological root – for example, child abuse or a broken family; still others may be a combination of all these factors.

However, traditional treatments often require drug therapy, which is expensive, and frequently responsible for dramatic side effects, including death. So it may be worth your while to first determine whether your problems or those of a loved one have been caused by an environmental agent that can be eliminated or safely controlled by neutralization-dosage therapy.

HYPERACTIVITY AND LEARNING DISABILITIES

There is no single definition of hyperactivity. One aspect of the disorder is an overly stimulated response that may show up as an inability to sit still, irritability, aggression, or moodiness. If you have a hyperactive child, you know it. You may not know the precise medical term, but you know you have a problem. Hyperactive children are into everything, fidgeting and restless; they may not have many friends, and they may pick fights with the few they do have. Or maybe they cry a lot. There is a good chance that they do not do well at school on any level. You may have been told that your hyperactive child is learning disabled or has "minimal brain dysfunction" (another name for the combination of hyperactivity and learning disabilities).

If you are like most parents of hyperactive children, you will probably do what Mary's parents did – take your child to a pediatrician or maybe to a neurologist. Like Mary, your child, if diagnosed as hyperactive, will probably be put on Ritalin, the appetite suppressant commonly prescribed for hyperactivity in children. It is not understood how an appetite suppressant works to quiet hyperactivity, but Ritalin and other common appetite suppressants from the amphetamine family, such as Dexedrine, are nevertheless the mode of therapy used by traditional physicians to treat hyperactivity. Not surprisingly, Ritalin causes a loss of appetite. This may be a desirable side effect for weight-conscious adults, but it can be very harmful for young children, who need to eat regularly to ensure proper growth and development.

Thorazine, the antipsychotic drug that produces a "functional lobotomy," is also used to treat hyperactivity in children. Of course, like any other potent drug, Thorazine is prescribed for children in smaller amounts than those taken by adults. But you may think twice before giving your child any amount of a drug that may cause permanent brain damage, tardive dyskinesia, or Parkinson's disease. Thinking twice may be especially appropriate when the alternative may be as simple and innocuous as the removal of certain foods or chemicals from your child's environment.

ONE DOCTOR'S EXPERIENCE   Dr. Doris Rapp, who has been a pediatric allergist since 1960, has spent the past eleven years studying the relationship between children's behavior and environmental allergies. She has found that these allergies can be responsible for a wide variety of symptoms – depression, for example:

> I can remember one little boy, Robbie, who, according to his mother, had never really smiled. She had pictures of him at birthday parties and things like that, and he was always down. He just had never smiled. She placed him on the diet, and within one week he was smiling.
>
> He mentioned that before, he used to be so sad that he wanted to put a knife "right here." We have a video of him wanting to put the knife in his chest.
>
> We have seen youngsters become very withdrawn and untouchable on damp days. They will write notes, for example, that nobody likes them, they don't deserve to be thanked, they don't deserve to be liked because they are not good. They tend to crawl under the furniture, and if you go to touch them, they pull away. Sometimes they will even put their hair in front of their face. No one can go near them.
>
> Then when we skin test them in the office and they don't know what they are being tested for, their behavior is exactly the same. And they're being tested for molds. When we give them the correct solution, on their own they walk over to their mother and give her a big hug and a kiss and say they love their mother.
>
> There is one eight-year-old that I saw today who becomes depressed and suicidal each year during the tree pollen season. Last year when she came in, she drew pictures which were very unhappy with sad faces. Then after we treated her for tree pollen, she drew a smiling face of a youngster who was very happy.[11]

Children suffering from the tension-fatigue syndrome may become totally exhausted after eating an allergenic food. Dr. Rapp says that she has seen children who eat peanut butter routinely for breakfast become so tired by the time they get to school that they can hardly hold their heads up. When they are food tested, they are found to be allergic to peanuts. When given the correct neutralization dosage of allergy peanut extract, the children become alert and are able to do their work in the morning.

Dr. Rapp says that other tension-fatigue children get "clingy – they sort of hang on the parents, and the parents say they have to be 'peeled off.' The child just whines and fusses and lies all over their mother."[12]

Many of these children exhibit changes in their handwriting, which goes right along with how they feel. Dr. Rapp explains that:

> The child who is exuberant and all over the place writes in a very large manner. However the writing may be upside down or backward or in mirror image. But the child who is depressed and goes into the corner frequently writes in *extremely* small letters. The writing will be as small as you can make it, or they will just write their name as a dot. Then when you treat them with the correct dilution of the stock allergy extract to which they are sensitive, then they can write in a normal fashion, and they act in a normal fashion.[13]

Although Dr. Rapp does not herself treat juvenile delinquent children, she says that based upon her experience with younger children, it is not difficult to see the role that food allergies may play in criminal behavior. Dr. Rapp gives examples of behavior linked to environmental allergies that, if untreated at an early age, could conceivably lead to criminal acts at a later date:

> The new patient that I saw today is a four-and-a-half-year-old boy. The mother brought him in because about two months ago he started to have these Dr. Jekyll–Mr. Hyde episodes. Many times he would become violent. He would take a knife, and he'd push the knife violently into a garbage bag. He tried to cut his hand, and he came at his father and said "I want to kill you."
>
> I have seen four-and five-year-olds, for example, who are not allowed to play with any of the neighbors in the street because they ride over the neighbor child. They don't take the baseball bat and hit the ball – they take the baseball bat and hit the neighbor.
>
> Some of these children are extremely aggressive. Many of them are destructive.[14]

Speaking of the nine-year-old who became vulgar each time he went to school, Dr. Rapp says that she has videos of a "very nice, intelligent youngster who draws very complicated pictures of fish and if you just inject a drop of this in his arm, within a short period of time he is vulgar and abusive, writing on the walls, jumping on the top of the furniture, giving everyone the finger. If you ask him to draw at that time he draws a note where he says somebody 'sucks royal.' He uses all the four-letter words, and he's just terrible."[15]

Dr. Rapp says that the extract of school air affects an area of the boy's brain, which makes him vulgar. When he is given the proper dilution, he's back to normal.

> In a few minutes he's drawing a fish again. On one occasion I said "C'mon, I'd like to hear you say some dirty words now." He looked at me some-

what startled and said, "Why do you want me to do that? I don't feel like it." Finally with a lot of prodding he said a couple of dirty words, but he didn't say it as if he meant it, whereas before he was having a great time, he was amused by his actions. And one has to wonder what type of individual he will become later on.[16]

Dr. Rapp says that many of these children batter their parents. We hear about wife-battering and child abuse, but most of us have never heard of parents being abused. Dr. Rapp says that some children hit and pinch their mothers repeatedly when they eat the wrong foods. She tells of a ten-year-old boy who hits his mother on the head with a soda-pop bottle when she is asleep.

It is not difficult to imagine what would happen if a child who talks vulgarly and tries to stab his father or hits his mother in the head while she is sleeping were eighteen years old and had an allergic reaction in public with no one to restrain him or her. These acts, uncontrollable and therefore often overlooked in a child, could easily foreshadow later criminal behavior.

Dr. Rapp agrees that this type of conduct could lead to criminal behavior at a later date. "These children are mean and nasty, some of them," she says.

Food or chemical reactions can also lead to depression and suicidal tendencies, both of which are forms of internalized violence – violence to the self.

Dr. Rapp recalls the case of "one little boy who was 12 ... who said to his mother that he had tried to kill himself several times by putting a pillow on his face, and he said, "each time I was chicken, and I had to take the pillow off."

And I can remember Beth – if she smells a chemical odor – for example, she used to use nail polish – and when the odor got to her, she would go out and sit in the middle of the street, hoping that the cars would hit her. Other times she would go into the bathroom and threaten to kill herself. That was at the age of fifteen. At the age of twenty-five, no one would be around to stop her. Would she go into the bathroom and kill herself? She'd be able to do it at that point.[17]

The symptoms of allergic reactions are so varied that it is impossible to list them. Below Dr. Rapp gives other examples of the types of symptoms that can be associated with environmental allergies. These are not the only types of allergic symptoms there are but illustrate a few of the many different ways that allergies may affect us.

One of the major distinctions between clinical ecology and traditional medicine is the emphasis clinical ecology places on an individualized approach to medicine. Each of us will react differently to our environment, and the way that we manifest our reactions is also individual.

Environmental allergies may cause extreme skin sensitivity or silly behavior. Some young children will take off all their clothes and refuse to put them back on. They don't want things touching their skin. According to Dr. Rapp,

> Silly or inappropriate behavior is another thing we see. We have a video of a fifteen-year-old boy who was thrown out of school at the age of twelve because he took his shirt off in school and wouldn't put it back on, which made me think of the younger children who take their clothes off and won't put them back on.
>
> I brought this young man in. He was on 60 mg of Ritalin a day, which is an extremely high dose. He went on the diet in the book and improved dramatically. After a period of a month or so he was off the Ritalin.
>
> I wanted to do some food testing. I put three drops of food coloring – you know, the French's or McCormick's food colorings that they use to color cakes or cookies; that sort – put the three drops under his tongue, and within about ten minutes, he's racing a car up his mother's leg going *wroom.* He would stop it just short of her chin. And then *wroom* ....
> Then at one point he put a car on top of his head and a sort of plastic airplane in his mouth, and he was trying to blow the airplane across the room. Then he got a giggling spell, which he said was better than marijuana or something like that. When I gave him the right dilution of the food coloring, he came right back to normal. You can see it's almost like a snap. He was all of a sudden a fifteen-year-old boy who was sensible and alert. He said that after he had been on the diet for a week, it was the first time that he could read the newspaper without Ritalin. Prior to that when he read, the words were all over the page.
>
> This youngster's life may be totally ruined by this experience. His allergies were not diagnosed early. He was very allergic to sugar as well as food coloring and he never did finish his education. He went into the service and had problems. He couldn't hold a job. Because he was unable to attain his education at the proper time, he ran into many problems, and he may have problems for the rest of his life. You have twelve years in which to get your education. If you are unable to do so in that period of time, it's hard to catch up when you're twenty.[18]

THE FOOD VERSUS DRUG CONTROVERSY   According to Dr. Randolph, hyperactivity and related syndromes are a growing problem in the United States. Rather than dealing with this problem at the level of environmental causation, orthodox medicine prefers to perpetuate the problem through the use of drugs. Of the 750,000 children seen for minimal brain dysfunction in 1978, 212,000 were put on medication and about 75 percent of them, or nearly 120,000 on methylphenidate hydrochloride [Ritalin].[19]

During the 1970s more than 100 million Ritalin tablets were prescribed for hyperactive children. The use of Ritalin became so widespread that a 1971 *Washington Post* article reported that some three to six thousand elementary school children in Omaha, Nebraska, were receiving amphetamines to modify their behavior. This report sparked such a controversy that a Senate subcommittee decided to investigate the matter. It reported alarm at the ease with which amphetamine prescriptions for children were available. The subcommittee found that often doctors merely acted as scribes, filling out prescriptions for the Ritalin based on a note from a parent or teacher without ever actually examining the child.[20]

A special Health, Education, and Welfare committee, formed to further investigate the problem, issued recommendations that barred anyone other than a physician from diagnosing and prescribing treatments. It forbade the pharmaceutical companies from promoting the use of the amphetamines for hyperactivity through any channels other than the normal medical ones, and it warned parents against being coerced into using this mode of treatment.

The use of Ritalin in the treatment of hyperactivity is still pervasive. Some researchers feel that the marked increase in childhood hyperactivity nationwide coincided with an increase in the amount of food additives in the diets of the typical American child. If a child is allergic to the additives, as was the fifteen-year-old who became silly when tested for food colorings, then a direct causal link can be clinically established between the behavior and the additive. When it is introduced, the child reacts, and when it is withdrawn or the correct neutralization dosage is administered, the symptoms go away.

Benjamin Feingold, M.D., in his book *Why Your Child is Hyperactive*,[21] was the first to bring to the attention of the American public the link between food additives and hyperactivity in children. Dr. Feingold found that foods eaten by children, such as Kool-Aid, candy, cakes, soft drinks, Jell-O, and luncheon meats, were among those containing the largest amounts of food additives. These substances build up in the body. Dr. Feingold found that when a child's body weight is taken into account, the amount of artificial dyes, flavors, and natural salicylates in their bodies at any given time can be substantial – substantial enough to cause hyperactivity.

Many clinical ecologists believe that studies were sponsored by the pharmaceutical industry and the food lobbyists to invalidate the findings of Dr. Feingold and others because of their vested interests. However, their studies, which showed no relationship between chemical additives and behavioral disorders, administered only 26 milligrams of food dye per day to the subjects, far less than the normal daily intake of the average six-to-ten-year-old. On the other hand, studies administering 100 to 150 milligrams of food dye per day did show significant behavioral changes in children at intervals of one, one-and-a-half, and three-hour intervals.[22]

Dr. Randolph writes, "Labeling a hyperactive child as in need of drugs eliminates the necessity of discovering the underlying problem which is causing his/her behavioral problems. While the psychologist probably had in mind psychological causes, the same can be said, even more emphatically, about the chemical and environmental causes of this disorder."[23]

Dr. Rapp gives two examples of how children react to sugar:

I brought in two children. One was a three-year-old boy, and the other a seven-year-old boy. Both of them ate, over half an hour, eight sugar cubes. The younger one had a classical temper tantrum, was throwing things all over, refused to draw or write. Then we gave him the correct dose of the cane sugar, and he was normal in about ten minutes.

The other boy, when he ate the sugar, the first thing that happened was that he got a headache. Then his bladder went into spasm, and he had to run to the bathroom. Then when he came back, he crawled under the furniture, which many of them do. They crawl in a dark corner, and when his mother came near, he tried to hit her. When we tried to get him to write his name, he was throwing the pencil and the pad all over the place. The nurse eventually had to crawl under the table to give him his next dilution of the sugar extract. His ears and cheeks became violently red during the reaction. Then when we gave him the right dilution of sugar, he was back to normal – writing, conversing, and being an extremely pleasant and nice boy.[24]

Just as the drug companies' studies exculpated food additives, articles are appearing in the medical literature asserting that sugar does not cause changes in children's behavior. Dr. Rapp says that in these studies the sugar was mixed in lemonade or juice and given to children after they had eaten, making it impossible to know what was going on.

Psychiatrists, allergists, and pediatricians who know the importance of food and chemicals for hyperactivity and other behavioral problems will immediately remove sugar and artificial ingredients from a patient's diet. Children so treated become markedly calmer within a brief period of time.

DEVASTATING AND LIFELONG EFFECTS Diagnoses of "hyperactivity" and "minimal brain dysfunction" can have lifelong repercussions on children. If they remain untreated, they can have problems in school, both socially and academically. They may never really fit into society, and they may be troublemakers and drop out of school. If you are a parent of a hyperactive child, you may have to spend a fortune on special tutoring and classes for your child. Even if the hyperactive child is treated by conventional means, he or she most likely will not be cured, and the long-term effects of amphetamine use by children is not yet determined. Even with Ritalin, hyperactive children may always feel like misfits, knowing that at any moment they may "flip out" if they stop taking the drug.

Clinical ecology may offer hope for hyperactive children and their parents. Dr. Rapp is careful to stress that allergic reactions are not necessarily responsible for all hyperactivity in children. Other factors may be the primary cause that are present in addition to the allergies. But in Dr. Rapp's experience, the hyperactive child is often an allergic child whose symptoms can be eliminated by proper diet, avoidance of the offending food(s), and neutralization-dosage therapy. With respect to these children, she says: "We have to make at least the people with young children aware that this problem can be helped. They don't have to learn to live with it. There are things that they can do themselves to try to recognize this problem and help their doctor to become more aware of it."[25]

Lendon Smith, M.D., of Portland, Oregon, known as "the children's doctor" from television, estimates that 70 percent of prisoners were hyperactive kids.[26]

One California probation department decided to do something about this common problem. They replaced the regular diet in their juvenile hall with a diet prescribed by Dr. Feingold, a diet that avoids sugar and food additives. Summarizing the results of this program, the chief probation officer writes: "Children, staff, school teachers, and parents all report less hyperactivity in youngsters who participate in the program . . . . In the past two years a remarkable difference has been observed in the behavior of inmates in the Tehama County Juvenile Hall. Additionally, children are receiving a more nutritionally sound diet and are learning to recognize how their feelings change with diet modification.[27] An additional bonus to the new dietary regimen was that the institutional food costs decreased by 14 percent.

Clinical ecologist William G. Crook, M.D., author of *The Yeast Connection* and a longtime advocate of environmental testing for food allergies, hyperactivity, and minimal brain dysfunction, comments: "The more we increase the awareness of the public and the medical profession about this, the sooner we'll have a lot of people feeling much better about themselves and everyone else. Before you label your child as a 'nervous child,' or a 'hyperkinetic child,' or a 'child with minimal brain dysfunction or dyslexia,' make sure that allergy, the great masquerader, isn't responsible for his problems."[28]

CRIMINAL BEHAVIOR AND ALLERGIES

The examples of hyperactive children given above show the fineness of the line between hyperactivity in children and criminal behavior. In many cases the only distinction may be whether the hyperactivity is diagnosed and treated at an age early enough to thwart irreparable damage done to the child by his or her antisocial behavior and learning impairments.

For decades now many criminologists have been attributing criminal juvenile delinquent behavior solely to sociological factors. In fact, one of the most important factors may be sociological, but not in the traditional sense. Poor and underprivileged children are often malnourished, either because of a lack of food or because of the non-nutritious and unhealthy nature of that food. These children are often brought up in single-mother households in which the mother herself may be taking drugs. The mother may work all day, leaving the children in the morning and returning to them late in the evening. In circumstances such as these, a mother may never notice that her child is acting strangely or doing poorly at school. She may consider a violent, aggressive attitude normal, given the lamentable circumstances in which she and her children live. Even if she does notice and does want to do something about it, chances are that she has neither the means to attain nor access to the proper kind of medical attention. Factors such as these are indeed sociological, but in the case of an allergic or malnourished child they may be compounded or caused by physiological factors.

Fortunately there is a small but growing number of mental health and criminal justice professionals who, recognizing the link between crime and diet, have been doing important work to get at the root of the crime problem that is currently plaguing this nation and ruining the lives of millions of Americans – perpetrators and victims alike.

The examples given by Dr. Rapp have shown that antisocial and violent behavior may begin at a very young age. Dr. Rapp has also shown that in many cases the cause of this behavior can be traced to a food allergy that triggers the behavior and that the behavior can be turned off when the correct neutralization dosage is given or the allergenic food eliminated from the diet of the child. Other clinical ecologists, such as Dr. Philpott, have shown that behavior ranging from mild irritability to full-blown psychosis may be triggered in adults by food allergies.

In addition to the work by clinical ecologists concerning the connection between environmental allergies and behavior, studies have been done within the criminal justice system on the role played by diet in criminal behavior.

THE SCHOENTHALLER STUDIES   In 1977 criminologists were sharply divided about whether human nutrition could affect behavior. The U.S. Senate Hearings on Human Nutrition stated that reporting on the topic was inconclusive and that the studies done to date did not meet their rigorous requirements.

As a result of these hearings, Steven Schoenthaller, Ph.D., coordinator of criminal justice at California State University at Stanislaus began a series of three studies at the Virginia Department of Corrections. The first study lasted seven months and involved fifty-eight juveniles who were detained in a juvenile detention facility. These youths ranged from runaways and battered children to those who had committed serious crimes. In his first study Dr. Schoenthaller removed refined sugar and, as much as possible, all foods and drinks containing refined sugar from the diets of these youths. Fruit juices replaced soda pop, and honey and molasses replaced jams, jellies, and sugar on their tables. Canned fruits were either packed in their own juices or rinsed of their packing syrup. Seven days after the changes had been implemented, changes in behavior were measured. Antisocial and aggressive behavior were reduced by a half, simply by lowering the consumption of refined sugar.[29]

Dr. Schoenthaller's second study was much more extensive than the first. It lasted two years and involved 276 juveniles. Again, antisocial behavior was shown to be reduced by half; rearrest rates were also half of what they had been. Violent crimes committed fell by 88 percent.[30]

These studies offered the first concrete link between diet and criminal behavior. The Virginia Department of Corrections was so impressed by the results that it permanently adopted the dietary changes instituted by Dr. Schoenthaller. Many other states have followed Virginia's example.

SCHAUSS'S RESEARCH Dr. Alexander Schauss, director of the Institute for Biosocial Research in Tacoma, Washington, has also done work showing the relationship between diet and behavior. In *Diet, Crime and Delinquency* he cites a program at the Alameda County Probation Department that watches over approximately 350 juvenile delinquents at youth camps, juvenile detention centers, and a dependent child-care facility. The department provided all its charges with a healthier diet while drastically reducing their sugar and refined-carbohydrate intake. Alameda's director of special services commented that the juveniles were "quieter and less rambunctious."[31]

According to Dr. Schauss's research, these youngsters are generally very interested in volunteering for programs involving biochemical workups. They want to understand the causes of their behavioral problems, and they show very little resistance to having their metabolism and brain chemistry evaluated. They generally accept changes in dietary regimen and supplementation.[32] As I shall explain below, the resistance comes from the professionals operating these institutions.

Another instance cited by Dr. Schauss was at the U.S. Naval Correctional Center in Seattle, Washington. The prison administrator, Chief Warrant Officer Gene Baker, curtailed the availability of refined carbohydrates for the inmates. In cooperation with his head cook, he reduced their intake of white flour and sugar. After a few months flour and sugar were removed altogether from the inmates' diets. They were allowed only a teaspoonful of sugar in their coffee or tea per day. The institution's medical log revealed a definite decrease in attendance at sick call, and that disciplinary reports were down 12 percent from the previous year.[33]

In 1979 the San Luis Obispo Juvenile Probation Department in California was awarded a one-year grant to establish a clinical ecology treatment program for difficult juvenile offenders. Dr. Schauss's staff conducted a thorough biochemical and nutritional analysis on each child, which showed that "all of the first juveniles handled by the program had significant body chemistry imbalances. The children were subject to environmental and food allergies which were negatively affecting their physiological and psychological processes.[34]

The juveniles' problems were treated through dietary change. Their families were encouraged to become part of this process. Nutrition classes were held to reeducate parents and children, and the child's home environment was investigated as a possible site of dietary or environmental allergens.

SUGAR AND MILK In the San Luis Obispo study, Dr. Schauss found that milk produced allergic symptoms typifying criminal behavior in almost 90 percent of the juveniles studied.[35] This observation coincides with studies made by other clinical ecologists that show milk to be responsible for a wide range of allergy-related symptoms in patients. Dr. Philpott, for example, found that 51 percent of his schizophrenic patients exhibited symptoms when tested for milk.[36] One explanation for the high rate of allergic reactions to milk may be the body's inability to break down many of the amino acids found in milk. We noted in Chapter 1 that an inability to digest foods properly may cause undigested protein molecules to enter the bloodstream, causing an allergic reaction as antibodies to these molecules are made.

Blood sugar disorders may also be a major culprit in antisocial behavior. Researchers have demonstrated that high blood sugar can cause many behavioral symptoms, including antisocial behavior, depression, and hyperactivity. As sugar consumption increases, so does concern for its effects on behavior and health.

As far back as 1979 the American Public Health Association concluded that the overconsumption of nonnutritious foods is a major health problem. Children who substitute snack and processed foods for staples may develop hypoglycemia, obesity, and degenerative diseases, such as cardiovascular disorders.

This knowledge has been circulating for some time among medical and lay communities, yet little attention has been paid to the sugar consumption of juveniles in correctional programs. Criminologists like Dr. Schoenthaller and Dr. Schauss are concerned about the consequences of this dietary inattention.

As Dr. Schauss writes, "In countless numbers of prisons, jails, and detention centers, I have observed the availability of coffee, sugar, candies, and sweet drinks for confinees. In some institutions, the quantities of these substances is limitless. Little or no interest is shown in treating suspected hypoglycemia among offenders [averaging 80 to 85 percent], yet most correctional facility medical personnel still treat the problem as nonexistent. The usual response is to prescribe medication when a delinquent or prisoner complains about dizziness, cold sweats, nervousness, and fatigue – all potential signs of hypoglycemia."[38]

We spoke with Dr. Schoenthaller in January 1987 and asked him to tell us about current work being done concerning diet and criminal behavior. He said:

> After all of the years of argument, we have discovered what the thing is all about. It looks like the problem is going to turn out to be nothing more complicated than low levels of malnutrition. To isolate the problem

we gathered data from fourteen institutions. Everyone was getting the same results. Kids were getting better slowly. Improvement was never sudden. It was a gradual thing.

Things like reactive hypoglycemia can be controlled in twenty minutes; IgE-mediated food intolerances take four or five days to clear up. We noticed that it took considerably longer with the kids in this [juvenile delinquent] group. We knew that hypoglycemia and IgE-mediated might be involved, but they were not the primary mechanisms here. We looked at the literature for illnesses that had slow recuperation, and the literature fit best with malnutrition. You take a malnourished person and you put them on a better diet, and they will improve gradually.[39]

Dr. Schoenthaller said that he had just finished a study of prison inmates in which their diets were supplemented with thiamin, niacin, zinc, and other essential vitamins and minerals. The result: "We found we could turn these institutions around," he said. "We found that we could get a 40 percent reduction in antisocial behavior in ten days."[40]

When asked about the link between allergies and juvenile delinquent behavior, Dr. Schoenthaller told us that as long ago as 1977 the head of School Food Nutrition Services in New York City decided that too much junk food was being served to children in public schools. A change was called for, and, according to Dr. Schoenthaller:

Some of my colleagues and I went in and analyzed academic performance in New York City public schools on the heels of these dietary changes. The New York City public schools use a standardized test called the California Achievement Test, as do schools all over the country. Every kid gets this test in grades one through eight. We needed to compare improvement in New York City public schools with any possible improvement in the rest of the country. The results of this study were released only thirty-five days ago.

Over four years, in 803 public schools, there was a 16 percent gain in academic performance ranking more than the average school range, on the heels of changes in the diet.

The diet involved the reduction of fat and sugar consumption, and they eliminated all foods that had synthetic food colors and synthetic food dyes. A couple of preservatives were removed as well.

Over the time span of the study the number of students in New York City public schools classfied as "learning disabled" dropped from 125,000 to 49,000. The definition of *learning disabled* is a student between grades two and nine who cannot do math or read within two grade levels of what he or she should have been able to do.

When you change the diet the way they did, by reducing the fat and sugar, you increase the nutrients per calorie. You are dealing with a sample that overall is probably getting enough calories but may not be getting enough nutrients. These changes probably just upped them in the right direction. It is unlikely that this many kids would be allergic to one of the items eliminated from the school diet, so we figured it had to be some underlying something across the board.

The study was written up in the *International Journal of Biosocial Research,* volume 8, number 2, January 1987.[41]

WHY ISN'T EVERYONE A CRIMINAL?   Many people wonder why two individuals who eat identically poor diets will not always end up with the same problems. For example, a guard may well eat the same junk food and drinks, the same soda and alcohol, as the prisoner he's guarding. So why aren't they both behind bars if diet really does influence behavior?

The answer is simple: Each person has his or her own biochemical individuality. We all react differently to the same elements in our environment, including the food we eat every day. The over-consumption of sugar by one individual may cause behavioral disturbances necessitating incarceration, while in another it causes a physiological imbalance leading to diabetes or heart disease. It is too often assumed that the lack of an obvious, immediate food or drug reaction means that we are not being negatively affected. But most individuals who are affected experience long-term, less obvious compounding effects. These effects must be dealt with and corrected sooner or later if we wish to live a long, disease-free life.

VITAMIN DEFICIENCIES   Dr. Philpott, in his private clinical psychiatric practice in Florida, has found that 53 percent of his patients are deficient in folic acid and 72 percent are deficient in vitamin B_6. Seventy-nine percent of his clients are deficient in one or more of the vitamins.[42] Dr. Philpott works not only with patients afflicted by mental disorders but also with victims of such physical maladies as diabetes. From clinical experience he found that two-thirds of initially noninsulin-dependent diabetics who have progressed to the use of insulin improved when treated by ecological principles.[43] In the next chapter I will show how some allergic symptoms are confused with other "physical" diseases.

ALLERGIES AND SWELLING OF THE BRAIN   In a 1977 editorial in *The Wall Street Journal* entitled "Can Chocolate Turn You Into a Criminal? ... Some Experts Say So," the author states, "An increasing number of scientists and physicians are concluding that malnutrition, food allergies and other nutritional deficiencies can set off aggressive and mind-warping behavior leading to criminal acts."[44]

Then, a psychiatrist is quoted as saying that "food allergies directly affect the body's nervous system by causing a noninflammatory swelling of the brain which can trigger aggression."[45] Yet despite studies at various correction centers that clearly show the connection between diet and behavior, little is being done to change dietary standards. Routine screening programs for food allergies and nutritional deficiencies in chronic offenders do not exist. Consequently, optimal health and rehabilitation are not being realized for more than 1 million confined juveniles and 300,000 prisoners detained each year.

RESISTANCE FROM THE MEDICAL AND LEGAL COMMUNITIES   Dr. Randolph believes that "the population as a whole could experience a tremendous increase in well-being and productivity if food and chemical susceptibility were routinely considered in each case of chronic disease, just as infection is today."[46]

Dr. Randolph accuses the medical establishment of classifying patients according to narrowly defined categories of diseases affecting either the physical or the emotional realm.

"Whatever the practical benefits of such a scheme," says Dr. Randolph, "it fails to describe these various complaints as part of an overall continuum of ill health in the life of each individual patient . . . . In actuality, ... most susceptible patients have a constellation of diseases, with few clear-cut distinctions between them."[47]

This opinion has been backed by reports and articles in major medical journals over the past fifty years. Yet as simple and powerful a concept as the nutrition-behavior link may be, it has met with much resistance in both the medical and legal communities.

Opponents claim that the researchers espousing such theories submit results that are invalid and lack credibility. These accusations paint a negative picture of innovative work currently being done by criminologists and clinical ecologists.

"With few exceptions," writes Dr. Schauss, "inmates are more willing to accept dietary changes than staff."[48] Dr. Schauss reports that even guards and staff members are more open to change than upper-level administration, who often commented to him that using nutrition to reduce the risk of an individual's reappearance in the criminal justice system was absurd.

Prison officials fear that an innovative approach may threaten or devalue their position within the existing system, and this makes it difficult to create change within these institutions. Sadly, they often even refuse to cooperate in important studies of ecological concepts because of the biases established by orthodox medicine.

A working alliance among criminologists, nutritionists, educators, and physicians is essential for further research into the role that biochemical individuality and nutrition play in antisocial and criminal behavior in children and adults.

We can play a vital role in that alliance, working to make society a safer and more harmonious place. With a tool as powerful as the ecological approach to mental illness and criminal behavior in our hands, can we afford not to raise our voices and answer the questions that our medical and legal communities seem reluctant to address?

If we don't, the cost may be dearer than life!

CHAPTER THREE

Allergy and Physical Health

HEADACHE AND ALLERGY

CASE ONE Sarah was a forty-year-old housewife with three children. One summer evening Sarah, her husband, and her children went over to a neighbor's house for a barbecue. The neighbor served the usual barbecue fare: hot dogs and hamburgers with all the trimmings, potato salad, chocolate cake, and ice cream. Sarah was in a particularly good mood. Her husband, Charlie, had at last gotten his long-deserved raise, and she was now going to be able to make the improvements on their house that she had had in mind for quite some time. Everyone was laughing and enjoying the summer evening. Without a thought Sarah helped herself to a second helping of everything: two hot dogs, extra potato salad, and another piece of cake. She wanted to have a good time and "forget" that these were precisely the foods that she suspected were linked to her migraine headaches.

On the way home she began to feel a little nauseous. By the time the family got home, Sarah had to be carried upstairs to her room. Her head was throbbing; her eyes were squinted to slits from the pain. Not until about 4 A.M. the following morning did she fall asleep from exhaustion.

Charlie had seen these migraines before, and they always terrified him. He couldn't stand seeing Sarah suffer, but he felt helpless. The family doctor had said that he couldn't do anything but prescribe a pain reliever.

Charlie had earlier overheard a fellow employee talking about a nutritional doctor who helped him with his migraines. Charlie was skeptical; he didn't believe in all that health-food stuff that everyone was talking about. But he was frantic – somebody had to help Sarah. The next day he got the name of the doctor, and he made an appointment for her for the following day. After hearing Sarah's history of migraines the doctor told Sarah that he suspected allergies to be at the root: allergies to meats treated with nitrates and to chocolate. Sarah groaned – hot dogs and sausage- and salami-type meats were her favorites. She ate them almost daily. She could pass on the beef, but she loved spicy cured meats. And chocolate... She underwent testing, and the doctor's suspicions proved correct. When he put drops of chocolate or nitrates under her tongue, her migraine syndrome started up. She also found that mustard had the same effect. The doctor put Sarah on a rotational diet and gave her drops of the neutralization dosage for each of these substances to relieve the symptoms in case Sarah indulged in these foods or ate them unknowingly.

CASE TWO   Alex was a top-notch investment banker; some considered him to be the top in his field. Years ago he had worked for one of the leading investment houses, but he found that he could make more money and was happier working on his own. For the previous ten years Alex had suffered from chronic migraines. His forehead was constantly wrinkled, and at times he looked as if he were wincing from the ever-present pain. Somehow Alex had learned to live with the pain. He used to take aspirin, but after a while they didn't help much unless he increased the dosage. Pain relievers prescribed by his doctor weren't much better. He was in such constant pain that he found that he couldn't enjoy food much anymore and was living primarily on milk and cheese together with fruits, vegetables, and some bread. He was conscious of his health and figured that this way he was at least getting the necessary protein and somewhat limiting the calories. Although Alex didn't overeat, he found that he was consistently putting on weight, to the point where he was thirty-five pounds overweight.

One day while reading Alex came across an article linking migraines to allergies. The article told of a simple, self-administered test called the Coca Pulse Test that could determine allergies and that often enabled people to eliminate their migraines as a result. Alex decided to try it. He felt a little silly; he didn't really see how allergies could cause his headaches since he never had asthma or hay fever or anything like that; but he didn't have much to lose.

The test consisted of placing a piece of food or a drop of liquid under his tongue first thing in the morning on an empty stomach. He had to take his pulse before he did this, then again thirty minutes afterward. During the thirty-minute period he had to remain still in order to avoid otherwise causing his pulse to rise. The test had to be done with pure food substances. For example, to test for an allergy to wheat, bread could not be used because it contains other substances such as yeast, sugar, oil, and salt. So to test for wheat, Alex had to place a wheat berry or wheat germ under his tongue. If after thirty minutes Alex's pulse rose by ten beats per minute, this was a good indication that he was allergic. So one day Alex tested for wheat. Nothing. The next day he tested for corn, putting a popcorn kernel under his tongue. Still nothing. The following day he tested for milk. Much to his surprise, his pulse rate increased by seventeen counts.

This got Alex to thinking. He decided to avoid milk for a while and see if just maybe there could be a connection. For the first few days he still had his headaches. He thought they let up for split-seconds at times, but he wasn't sure. Then on the morning of the fifth day, he awoke for the first time in ten years without a migraine. Alex has remained migraine free. As an unexpected bonus he also dropped fifty pounds without even dieting over the two years following the elimination of milk from his diet.

THE MYSTERIOUS HEADACHE   Sarah and Alex are two of the more than 25 million people who consult their physicians each year with the same complaint – headache. Although there are various types of headaches, about 50 percent of these people suffer from migraines, the most serious type. Dr. Claude Frazier refers to them as "perhaps the most mysterious of all headaches."[1]

Literally, *migraine* means "half head." Migraine sufferers, who make up about 20 percent of the population, usually experience pain on only one side of their heads. On the average their migraines occur about twice per month with no pain between attacks.

With millions of Americans suffering from migraines on a regular basis, what inroads has traditional medicine made in their treatment?

Very little. Unfortunately, most doctors tell their patients that there is nothing they can do about migraines except prescribe pain relievers to mask the pain. Americans spend more than $500 million annually on aspirin and other assorted pain relievers; much of this is taken in an attempt to relieve migraine headaches.

Yet Dr. Theron Randolph states, "There is no need for a person to suffer for years on end with persistent headaches when the cause of these disorders can often be identified and relieved by eliminating certain common substances from the environment."[2]

With sales of pain relievers totaling more than a half a billion dollars each year, pharmaceutical manufacturers have a vested interest in promoting their use. Pharmaceutical companies play a much larger role than most people suspect in the kind of treatment we receive for our medical problems. Advertising by drug companies often constitutes 25 to 50 percent of revenues of medical journals. These medical journals are the major source of continuing education for most physicians. In this author's opinion the amount of money spent on advertising gives the drug companies a position to dictate the types of articles that are published in medical publications. Editors of these publications are very well informed about what their major financial contributors will approve or disapprove of. Accordingly, most medical journals publish articles touting the efficacy of particular drugs and reinforcing notions concerning the incurable nature of many diseases. These journals almost consistently reject articles concerning treatments that are nutritional or dietary in nature since they represent a direct threat to the financial interests of the pharmaceutical companies. Many articles appear in medical publications that claim to disprove the benefits of a vitamin; or dietary changes are sponsored directly or indirectly by pharmaceutical companies. That is to say, a drug company may sponsor research which purports to be objective on vitamins but, the protocols are flawed and hence the results misleading. This certainly was the case with vitamin C and cancer. The amounts and duration of the research were far too low to be effective so they published articles saying vitamin C and E has no therapeutic value. Not so. At a very low dose it has no therapeutic value but at the level that medical nutritionists have been using those two vitamins have helped many patients. This may explain at least in part why clinical ecologists have difficulty in making such simple and inexpensive practices as elimination diets and neutralization therapy gain more acceptance in the medical community.

Clinical ecologists agree that headaches are not a disease but are often due to food or chemical sensitivities. The allergic headache may manifest itself exclusively as head pain, or it may be joined by such symptoms as nausea, vomiting, and diarrhea.

Although treatment is often as simple as following an elimination diet, traditional doctors frequently prescribe surgery or long-term medications that at best award only temporary relief while possibly creating further problems down the line.

No one claims to have a cure, but clinical ecologists are achieving encouraging results with their patients by correctly identifying and eliminating their allergens. For many, relief is obtained simply by isolating and eliminating common allergens from the environment and/or diet.

The allergy-headache link is not a new concept. In fact, more than fifty years ago, Albert Rowe, M.D., author of the first major work on allergy, *Food Allergy (Its Manifestations, Diagnosis and Treatment)*, stated, "Migraine is best explained as an allergic phenomenon, and food allergy in my experience is the most commonly recognized cause of this condition. Its manifestations vary in degree and may be associated with transient nervous complications."[3]

One of Dr. Rowe's patients experienced severe migraines for nearly twenty-five years; his headaches were accompanied by a lack of concentration, fatigue, weakness, nausea, and severe abdominal pain. The patient had needlessly undergone a tonsillectomy and nasal surgery in hopes of relieving his intense discomfort. His only true relief came from the elimination of wheat, dairy products, and eggs from his diet.

This case exemplifies how easily allergic symptoms are misdiagnosed and how much such a misdiagnosis costs the patient in unnecessary suffering. Nearly one-fifth of Dr. Rowe's patients had needlessly undergone surgery for relief of their headache symptoms before they were fortunate enough to fall into his care.

Sixty years ago, Dr. Rowe hypothesized, "Migraine resulting from food allergy is probably due to a localized swelling or vascular spasm in the brain. Pain in some cases ... has been so severe as to suggest brain tumor, and exploration has revealed swelling of the brain itself."[4]

Despite the strong evidence that Dr. Rowe and many of his colleagues have presented linking migraine and food allergy, physicians are still slow to accept this theory.

"This is due, in my mind," wrote Dr. Rowe, "to the fact that skin reactions to foods are often absent or difficult to interpret."[5] Skin tests for allergy don't work in these cases, he supposed, because the allergen is actually a metabolically altered form of the food, "the nature of which is unknown, and for which, therefore, no skin testing materials are available."[6]

MORE CLINICAL EVIDENCE   In a recent study of migraine using elimination diets, in which an average of ten common foods were avoided, subjects experienced a dramatic decline in the number of headaches per month. Eighty-five percent of those participating became headache free; twenty-five percent of the patients who were hypertensive (had high blood pressure) at the onset of the study once again had normal blood pressure when they followed an elimination diet.[7]

Another study one year later showed that migraine sufferers were allergic to an average of three food groups. When the offending foods were removed from the diet, headaches stopped within two weeks and patients became symptom free for the first time in years.[8]

ANATOMY OF A MIGRAINE   If you are a migraine sufferer, you may have found that your migraines are often preceded or accompanied by nausea, stomachaches, dizziness, or blurred vision. Because nausea and stomachaches are so often precursors of a migraine, many clinical ecologists believe that migraines are the result of a digestive difficulty. When digestion is not working properly, protein molecules may enter the bloodstream; the body reacts to this by making antibodies, causing the allergic reaction. This abdominal distress has also led some clinical ecologists to believe that migraines may be caused by allergic reactions in the stomach. These reactions then set into motion a chain of other reactions that culminate as a migraine.

The throbbing pain, nausea, dizziness, visual impairment, and other unpleasant symptoms that accompany a migraine headache are all part of the allergic response. The mechanism that causes migraines is so far unclear, but as Dr. Randolph puts it, "The physical manner in which allergies cause headache is not entirely known, nor is this information crucial to either patient or physician."[9]

Because a migraine does not always occur until sometime after you have eaten a food to which you are allergic, it may be difficult for you to make a connection between your diet and your migraines.

To complicate matters further, if the food or chemical that causes your migraine is part of an addictive-allergic reaction, you may find that your migraine is at first relieved after you eat the offending food. Or in the case of a cyclic allergy, you may only get a migraine following frequent consumption of the food. If you eat the food only on rare occasions, it may not bring on an allergic reaction, and you may never suspect it of being responsible for your headaches.

If you are under stress, it may also contribute to your migraines. Any sort of stress – physical stress from an illness, poor diet, cigarettes, or tobacco; emotional stress from a job or a strained relationship – any type of stress can play a role both in bringing on the migraine itself and in weakening the body and thereby increasing its susceptibility to allergies.

If you are particularly stressed for a prolonged period of time, you may even develop sensitivities to chemicals secreted in the body when it is under stress. These chemicals, through the allergic process, may also cause migraines.

It is for this reason that I always recommend that migraine sufferers practice stress reduction as well as eliminate allergens from their environment. Any form of relaxation that works for you is fine. It can be a sauna, a calm walk, meditation, a hot bath, or whatever else relaxes and soothes you, provided that you do it on a fairly regular basis.

WOMEN MORE SUSCEPTIBLE   Statistics show that twice as many women as men suffer from migraine.

Dr. Ellen Grant, a British researcher, offers an explanation: "The large cyclic change in tissue enzymes in women ... may help to explain why women have more overt reactions to food and chemicals premenstrually and why they are more likely to have migraines than men."[10]

Although the medical evidence is not yet complete, the toxic effects of oral contraceptives have been implicated as well. Their usage seems to produce severe migraines and multiple food allergies in women susceptible to allergies. The potentially serious side effects are one reason for avoiding this means of birth control.

MIGRAINE IN CHILDREN Although we usually associate migraines with high-stress adult life, "migraine in the early years of life is commoner than is generally supposed."[11]

Migraine headaches are not uncommon in childhood, even as early as infancy. One study in the 1950s involved fifty clinical cases that included only children ages six and up, most between nine and twelve. Although the onset of migraine occurs most frequently in young adulthood, about 30 percent of migraine sufferers manifest symptoms before age ten.[12]

It's not uncommon for children of five years or younger to be seen by a doctor for allergic conditions such as asthma and to have a secondary condition of migraine diagnosed. This diagnosis is usually made only after a detailed case history is taken.

Heredity is certainly a factor. Some physicians have reported that in as many as 85 percent of their pediatric patients, at least one parent, grandparent, or sibling had migraines. However, clinical ecologists warn that although a personal or family history of allergy is suggestive, it is not conclusive evidence of a migraine's origin. A history of allergy means that it is *more likely* to be a factor in the migraine, but a negative history by no means rules out allergy as a cause.[13]

Migraine symptoms in children are very similar to those in adults, but there are some differences. Preheadache symptoms in children include lethargy, loss of appetite, and abdominal discomfort. Adults commonly experience irritability and abdominal hunger beforehand.

Fevers of as high as 104 degrees Fahrenheit may occur during a childhood migraine. According to Jerome Glaser, M.D., "Since this does not occur in the adult, the presence of fever may draw attention away from the diagnosis of migraine to an explanation of the subsequent abdominal pain, nausea, and vomiting as heralding the onset of an acute infection. Acute appendicitis may be suspected."[14]

All these allergic symptoms, including abdominal distress, vertigo, fever, anxiety, and sweating, are easy to misdiagnose.

Preheadache symptoms and migraine attacks are of shorter duration in children than in adults. However, nausea is more intense in the youngsters, and the frequency of the attacks is much greater. It is not uncommon for a child to experience two or three attacks in one week. For most, the headache usually lasts an average of two hours, but it can continue for as long as eighteen hours in some cases.

As an allergic child gets older, the abdominal discomfort decreases while the headaches intensify. At approximately twelve years of age, symptoms become like those of adults.

Parents report that children suffering from migraine are sensitive, nervous, and of uneven temperament, with various behavior disturbances. Attacks can be brought on by nervous tension, insufficient sleep, irregular meals, fatigue, exposure to bright sunlight, and watching motion pictures. Even if migraines are of allergic origin, psychic stimuli can instigate an attack.

One can only imagine how unrestricted hours of television viewing and video games may affect sensitive children.

DOES YOUR CHILD HAVE ALLERGIC HEADACHE? Many parents are naturally concerned about determining whether their child suffers from allergic headaches, particularly if the child is too young to articulate a complaint. Pediatricians suggest that the following signs may indicate that your child or toddler is experiencing an attack: wrinkling of the forehead, restlessness, holding or rubbing of the head, and crying.[15]

Physicians specializing in the allergic child have found that in most cases in which the migraine was proven due to food allergy, the offending foods were discovered not by skin tests but by elimination diets.

DIET IS THE ANSWER A recent double-blind study published in *Lancet* showed that out of eighty-eight children with severe and frequent migraines, 93 percent recovered after following elimination diets.[16] The associated allergic symptoms exhibited by these children – such as abdominal distress, asthma, eczema, and behavioral disorders – also improved. For the majority of those in whom migraine was provoked by nonspecific factors, such as extreme temperatures, fatigue, flashing lights, or blows to the head, this provocation ceased to trigger headaches while the children adhered to the allergy-free diet. This was possibly due to a rebalancing of the body's chemistry. The better the internal health, the easier it is to offset or resist external toxins or trauma.

The researchers conducting this important study concluded, "This trial shows that most children with severe frequent migraine recover on an appropriate diet, and that so many foods can provoke attacks that any food or combination of foods may be the cause."[17]

Clinical ecologists stress that it is essential for allergic children to avoid *all* offending foods in their diets.

Drs. J. Egger, J. Wilson, J. F. Soothill, et al., stated in the *Lancet* article, "If a patient avoids only some of the foods that provoke symptoms, he/she may eat more of other provoking foods and so have worse symptoms."[18] This holds true for the mere avoidance of food colors and additives in your children's diet. Although these ingredients may be the underlying cause of migraines in some individuals, they may not be the only culprits. A child who is allergic to food coloring and is also allergic to milk will not benefit from eating all-natural vanilla pudding. He will still react to the milk. This is one of the shortcomings of the Feingold diet, in which only food additives and refined sugar are eliminated. Although the impact of this diet cannot be denied, it does not cover all the bases for a food-intolerant child.

DIAGNOSIS AND TREATMENT The diagnosis of an allergic migraine is based upon several findings, including a family and personal history of migraine attacks and known allergy symptoms.

Difficulty may arise in diagnosis if a food allergen evokes a slow response. In these cases an accurate diagnosis may require taking large amounts of the offending substance over a period of several days before an allergic headache is triggered.

Treatment of an allergic headache involves rest, the complete elimination of *all* allergens, neutralization-dosage therapy, and the removal of focal or localized infections – e.g., in the ear, nose, or throat – to rebalance the immune and other systems.

The sensitive person must also keep in mind that *new allergies to different foods may develop* and that sensitization may vary over time for each individual.

A cautionary note: Because each person is biochemically unique, there is no single diet beneficial for all headache sufferers.

Dr. Randolph warns in his book *An Alternative Approach to Allergies* that "since certain physicians have promoted alleged 'anti-headache diets,' it is important to emphasize … that there is no mass-applicable shortcut to controlling such painful syndromes. What affects one patient does not trouble the next. There is simply no substitute for working out one's own food allergy picture."[19]

MIGRAINES ARE NOT INCURABLE Contrary to what most migraine sufferers are being told, migraines are not incurable in most cases. If the root cause of the migraine is discovered, there is a good chance that future episodes can be avoided.

One way of getting at the root cause of your migraine is to go to a clinical ecologist who will prescribe an elimination diet for you based on your own personal case history. After four days to a week on that diet, you will be tested by the ecologist to determine the foods or substances to which you are allergic. After that, a rotational diet or neutralization therapy may be used to treat your migraines.

A less expensive way to diagnose your headaches could be the self-administered Coca Pulse Test described in the case of Alex. This test is particularly efficacious when you suspect that a particular substance may be causing you problems. If you suffer from cyclic or addictive allergies, you may not have any ideas to which food or substance you are allergic. In this case, seeing a qualified physician may be your only alternative.

Keep in mind, however, that we are often allergic to the foods that we consume the most frequently. Hence, even though, for example, you may not eat a lot of corn, you may cook with corn oil, eat margarine made from corn oil, and eat a lot of ready-made foods, many of which contain corn starch or corn syrup. You may thus be "abusing" corn without even knowing it. If you are going to do self-testing via the Coca Pulse Test, it is important to do a careful analysis of your diet.

NEUROSIS NOT THE CAUSE Dr. Rowe stated, "Every case of

migraine should be studied with the possibility of food allergy in mind. Many discussions of migraine lay most emphasis on neurosis as a cause. It is true that many of these sufferers are introspective, analytical, and neurotic. This is due in large measure, however, to their continued effort at self-help since all types of medical treatment have been of little benefit in the past. Allergy explains all the symptoms of migraine better than any other cause offered to date, and in my experience food allergy is the most probable type of sensitization operative in migraine."[20]

FATIGUE AND ALLERGY

CASE ONE Mike was in his midforties, married, with two children. Lately he had found that no matter how early he went to bed at night, he always awakened feeling tired and sluggish. He remembered that when he was a child he used to jump out of bed no later than seven, energized and enthusiastic about a new day. At that time, he couldn't imagine how anyone could sleep until ten o'clock. Now, if he wasn't awakened by his alarm clock, he could easily sleep until noon, even after going to bed at nine the night before.

Mike owned a successful clothing manufacturing company. He loved his work, but he found it exhausting. That was what frustrated him the most. He just didn't seem able to muster the energy to run the company the way he wanted to run it.

And then there was the family. He loved them all very much. He used to go out and shoot a few baskets with his son when he'd get home from work, or he'd help his daughter with her homework. He used to help his wife, Betty, prepare dinner and clean up afterward. Now all that seemed like a dream in which someone else played the central role. All he could do was come home and slump into his armchair, eat a little dinner, and start to get ready for bed.

Everything seemed to be falling apart. His clients complained that they weren't getting the attention they were used to, and some threatened to withdraw their business. Betty and the kids were mad at him because he didn't do anything with them anymore. In fact, just the other night, when Mike had cancelled a dinner party engagement because he was too tired, Betty had said that she was so fed up that she was thinking about a separation. "You used to be so much fun!" Betty screamed. "A real joy to be around. Now I feel like I don't even know you. You never want to do anything. You're always tired, and I'm fed up."

Mike decided that he had to do something. He went to the doctor for a physical and told the doctor to test him for everything. Nothing abnormal showed up. The doctor suggested that he go to a psychiatrist; maybe something was upsetting him psychologically. But Mike didn't buy that. He was happy with his life – his wife, his kids, his job. He didn't think his problem was psychological.

Mike had been "into health foods," as his friends said sarcastically, for some time. In some of those books he had read about the role that food allergies can play in the way one feels. He didn't give it much credance, however, and thought it was just another trend. But he believed in eliminating refined sugars and carbohydrates from his diet, and he avoided junk foods like commercial chips, cakes, and candies, as well as processed foods like processed cheese and luncheon meats. He ate a lot of salads, grains, and fruit and had almost eliminated meat from his diet. But the idea that foods like whole wheat or cheese, which had been around for hundreds of years, could cause his fatigue seemed ridiculous to him.

Nevertheless, he decided to go to see an environmental allergist, just in case. He was convinced that something had to work. The allergist took Mike's case history and asked for a detailed list of everything that Mike ate and drank. The doctor looked at the list and said there might be some sensitivity to wheat and dairy because Mike ate it every day. The doctor put Mike on an elimination diet and told Mike to stick to it religiously. "Remember," said the doctor, "nothing but the things on this list. No colas, coffee, tea, or alcohol." Mike cringed. He had forgotten to put coffee on his original list of things he ate and drank. He didn't drink much – only a cup of freshly ground French Roast in the morning and maybe two on the weekend. He didn't say anything to the doctor, but he decided to cut out coffee from his diet, too.

When he came back, the doctor tested him with drops of substances placed under his tongue. Mike didn't know what they were. He didn't experience much change for the most part. Every once in a while he felt a bout of drowsiness. But one substance toward the end made him feel that he was going to fall over with exhaustion. That was it. The doctor looked at Mike somewhat accusatorily. "I thought you weren't giving me the whole picture" he said. "That was coffee extract."

Mike was also found to be mildly allergic to milk and wheat and was put on a rotational diet for those products. Mike agreed to eliminate coffee altogether. As a result, Mike feels like a new person, or as Betty tells everyone, "He's back to being the fun-loving, energetic guy that I married."

CASE TWO   Ten-year-old Chris was driving everybody crazy. His parents, his teachers, and even his friends were fed up. One minute Chris would be fine; then all of a sudden, for no reason at all, he would get irritable, telling everyone to leave him alone and stop picking on him. A few minutes later, Chris would become lethargic and depressed. He didn't want to do anything. Often he'd tell his friends to go away, that he didn't want to play anymore. At school he would fall asleep in class, no matter how often his teachers chastized him. His parents found that he was having trouble concentrating; lately his grades had been going down.

At least Chris didn't throw the temper tantrums he used to throw as a child, in which he would bite and spit and attack people for no reason.

His mother, Amy, said that Chris didn't look right. His face was sallow, and he had dark circles under his eyes. Before, when he would throw the tantrums, his ears and cheeks would become bright, bright red. Now his cheeks became very flushed when he became irritable.

Chris's parents had taken him to doctors. At first he had been diagnosed as "hyperactive" and put on Ritalin. After the temper tantrums disappeared, everyone thought he was well. The only explanation the doctors could find for his lethargy was that he was in his formative years and needed his sleep. They suggested that he go to bed earlier at night. But his parents knew this was not the problem. They already had him in bed by eight o'clock. It just didn't make sense.

Amy decided to talk to her friend who studied health and nutrition to see if she had read anything about this type of thing in children. Amy's friend told her that she had just read an article on allergic tension-fatigue syndrome that she had just been going to call Amy herself because the article reminded her so much of Chris. The friend gave Amy the name of the doctor who had written the article, and even though the doctor's office was a good two-hour drive from their house, Amy made an appointment for Chris.

Much to Amy's surprise, the doctor, a pediatric allergist, was not surprised by Chris. She explained the tension-fatigue syndrome to Amy in greater detail than Amy's friend had, and she told Amy that it was often caused by food or chemical allergies.

After testing it was discovered that Chris's symptoms could be induced like clockwork by bananas, chocolate, and eggs. Once these foods were eliminated from Chris's diet, he was full of energy, his grades improved at school, and the dark circles under his eyes even went away.

OUR LACK OF NATURAL ENERGY   All of us experience fatigue at one time or another. It can be from staying up too late last night watching a Greta Garbo movie, or it may be because something was bothering you and you stayed up all night thinking about it. Or maybe, against your better judgment, you had a cup of coffee after dinner and were awake tossing and turning all night because of it.

I have a friend who has more energy than anyone I know. He's up, wide awake, at six in the morning, jogs, breakfasts, and is at work before eight. He accomplishes more than two regular people in the course of his workday and still has the energy to socialize almost every night. He rarely gets more than three to four hours of sleep a night and firmly believes that more is unnecessary.

Two months ago his father passed away. He handled all the funeral arrangements and took care of his mothers and sisters. In short, he took charge of the situation the way he normally does.

But for the last month he has been sleeping until noon, sometimes until midafternoon. The shock of his father's sudden death, all the responsibilities placed on him, and his own grief exhausted him. He keeps saying, "I can't believe that I need all this sleep." But he does need it. Emotional stress can be just as debilitating as strenuous exercise. Both body and mind need sleep to relax, to restore and heal themselves.

Maybe it is because feeling tired is seen as a normal response that excessive fatigue is not recognized as a medical problem. Yet if we took a look around, we see that many suffer from a sort of chronic fatigue that is far from normal.

Abundant natural energy is our strongest indicator of optimal well-being. This energy may ebb for short periods of time due to the types of stress mentioned above, but a prolonged, long-term lack of vitality is an indicator that something needs adjustment in your lifestyle. We all *deserve* enough energy both to enjoy and sustain personal relationships and to meet the day's challenges. Yet in today's frenzied and often polluted world, access to our wellspring of natural energy and enthusiasm may be blocked by environmental factors.

An increasing number of Americans have energy levels that are artificially elevated or depressed. Many feel that they just would not have the energy to get through the day without coffee or tea. After a day of artificial stimulation, they may feel simultaneously exhausted and wound up. Maybe an alcoholic drink will be "needed" to help them unwind, or a tranquilizer to help them sleep.

Natural energy and tranquility are increasingly rare. Many of us are caught up in a whirlwind lifestyle in which we feel that we can't function without caffeine to energize us and alcohol or tranquilizers to help us relax. But these are palliative measures, not solutions; they serve only to aggravate the underlying problem. Instead of resorting to such self-destructive measures, we should be examining our personal environment – our food and chemical intake and our lifestyles – to find the culprit behind our lack of natural energy.

THE TENSION-FATIGUE SYNDROME The tension-fatigue syndrome may affect many more Americans than is even suspected. All too often irritable behavior, fatigue, lethargy, and depression are attributed to solely psychological factors. Although the psyche certainly can play a role in these states, clinical ecologists are finding that a much larger proportion of them than we imagine are due to food allergies and diet.

The tension-fatigue syndrome can drastically decrease the quality of life of the sufferer. If you have this condition, you may wake up exhausted, drag yourself out of bed, and look forward to the day ahead with dread. Every so often you may ask yourself what happened, when it all changed for you. You remember all the energy and enthusiasm you had for life as a child, and you wonder where it went. You may not laugh much anymore; your primary concern may be just how you are going to manage to hold your head up for another day. This may lead to depression and even suicidal tendencies if you imagine the rest of your life will be so dreary. Most traditional physicians do not recognize symptoms like these as of physical origin and will probably send you off to a psychiatrist. The psychiatrist will probably look to your past and try to figure out what could have started all this, but he or she will not look for answers in the foods you have been eating for so long. If you are extremely tense, the psychiatrist may prescribe a tranquilizer, which will only aggravate the fatigue side of your symptoms. If you are really depressed, he or she may put you on other drugs.

Note that in the cases of Mike and Chris, the doctors never once thought to suspect a food allergy as the source of trouble. Doctors on the whole tend to view these symptoms as psychological or psychosomatic. They tend to prescribe drugs or other invasive therapy (like electroconvulsive therapy), when simple elimination and rotation diets could be the best treatment of all.

There are a number of reasons why the tension-fatigue syndrome is often misdiagnosed as psychosomatic. First, most traditional physicians fail to see or to acknowledge the link between diet and disease except in certain well-defined cases. This is especially true in the case of mental disease, where, for example, traditional medicine recognizes that a vitamin B_3 deficiency is the cause of pellagra, and that this disease, which causes symptoms of dementia (or psychosis) and death, can be cured by small quantities of the vitamin. Most doctors do not, however, recognize that megadoses of vitamins can play a significant role in the treatment of other mental disorders, such as hyperactivity in children and schizophrenia, even though numerous double-blind studies prove exactly that they can. Second, the symptoms of the tension-fatigue syndrome often resemble those of certain psychiatric disorders, so the physician treats them like those disorders. Based on the evidence provided by the clinical ecologists concerning the significant role played by diet in our behavior, it is likely that many people who were previously labeled manic depressive, schizophrenic, or hyperactive were in fact only suffering the symptoms of extreme food or chemical sensitivities.

A third reason that the tension-fatigue syndrome is so often misdiagnosed is that it frequently does not produce positive results in skin tests. In the intradermal test for instance, the allergen may not produce the *wheal* that usually appears when you are allergic to the allergy extract injected. Since the wheal is the only criterion considered by most traditional allergists, the allergy goes undetected. (I will discuss allergy tests in Chapter 5.)

A SHORT HISTORY   Information connecting the tension-fatigue syndrome to food and inhalant allergies has been available for over fifty years! In the 1930s the condition was described for the first time in the English medical literature by Dr. Rowe, who referred to it as "allergic toxemia."[21]

According to Dr. Rowe, this toxemia produced nervousness in allergic adults and children. Some of the symptoms he described were drowsiness, irritability, despondency, fatigue, weakness, bodily aching, and a feeling of "being poisoned."[22] Other contemporary reports described the syndrome, but they received as little attention and acceptance fifty years ago as they do today.

One positive and prophetic response to Dr. Rowe's article on allergic toxemia stated, "Allergy in general, and food allergy in particular, is assuming more and more importance in medicine as our understanding grows. There is no doubt in my mind that a certain group of patients complaining of an indefinite and obscure chain of symptoms such as those described by Dr. Rowe are suffering from food allergy."[23]

In the mid-1940s, Dr. Theron Randolph referred to this syndrome as "allergic fatigue" and described for the first time the facial pallor, swollen eyelids, and dark circles under the eyes associated with this disorder. He coined the term *brain-fag* for the more severe and debilitating form of mental fatigue experienced with this condition.[24]

Dr. Randolph writes, "Brain-fag is characterized by mental confusion, slowness of thought, lack of initiative and ambition, irritability, occasional loss of sex drive, despondency, as well as bodily fatigue, weakness and aching."[25]

Later, Frederick Speer, M.D., gave this disorder its present name. In a classic paper entitled "The Allergic Tension-Fatigue Syndrome,"

Dr. Speer wrote, "The impression given is that of a child who is torn between two extremes of feeling; at one extreme, over-reactivity or tension, at the other, under-reactivity or fatigue. Tension and fatigue occur in varying degrees in different patients, but both are present in virtually all cases."[26]

The mechanisms of the tension-fatigue syndrome are not fully known. It is believed, however, that the allergic reaction acts directly on the nervous system, causing characteristic behavioral and physical abnormalities.

Says Dr. Claude Frazier, "The mechanism of allergic tension-fatigue syndrome, like that of migraine, is open to speculation."[27]

SYMPTOMS   To summarize, the symptoms experienced in the tension-fatigue syndrome include:

- fatigue
- weakness
- lack of energy and ambition
- drowsiness
- mental sluggishness
- nightmares
- insomnia
- inability to concentrate
- bodily aches
- poor memory
- irritability
- fever
- chills and night sweats
- restlessness
- emotional instability

Sometimes these symptoms are accompanied by mild to severe mental depression, generalized muscular aches and pains (especially in the back of the neck, the back, and thigh muscles), swelling around the eyes, and increase in heart rate.

Discoloration in the eye region may appear and disappear on a daily basis or even throughout the same day, depending on the allergen exposure and subsequent response. This symptom is sometimes the only obvious sign of allergic reaction.

As I've emphasized before, allergy is an individualized disease. Two people may suffer from the same type of allergy, but it may not be caused by the same allergen, nor may the symptoms be identical. This is especially true in the case of the tension-fatigue syndrome. You may suffer from tension-fatigue due to an allergy to wheat. Your symptoms may be chronic fatigue, depression, and headache. Your best friend may also have the same syndrome due to allergies to milk and chocolate. His or her symptoms may be extreme nervousness, irritability, confusion, and inability to concentrate.

If, for example, you experience a brain allergy when eating wheat, then your symptoms may include lethargy, confusion, and depression. If your allergy is vascular (of the blood vessels), then it may be responsible for your high blood pressure and heart palpitations. If it is gastrointestinal, you may have nausea, gas, diarrhea, or digestive difficulties.

ONSET AND DURATION   The tension-fatigue syndrome can occur at any age. Documented cases range from infants to persons in their seventies. The duration ranges from several months to several decades. In some adults, the extreme fatigue, body aches, and depression interfere with work and domestic life. As the tension attacks increase in frequency, the fatigue symptoms are likely to persist continuously between episodes. It is not uncommon for fatigue to be the allergic individual's major complaint.

SLEEP DOESN'T HELP   If you suffer from the tension-fatigue syndrome, you may find that sleep does not relieve the fatigue. Even if you go to bed early, you may find it difficult to get out of bed in the morning. It is not unheard of for allergic people to sleep for up to fifteen hours for several consecutive nights in an attempt to overcome their fatigue, only to find that they are still tired.

The tension-fatigue syndrome often goes hand in hand with addictive allergies. People who are exhausted and irritable in the morning may be suffering from an addictive allergy. After not eating, drinking, or smoking during the night, they awake in the morning with withdrawal symptoms. Once they have their morning coffee, cigarette, or eggs on wheat toast, the symptoms go away – until they begin to experience withdrawal again.

By their very nature addictive allergies are masked. The food seems to be doing you well; it seems to give you energy. In fact its long-term effect may be to rob you of your natural energy and vitality. The long-term effects of this artificial stimulation followed by exhaustion are extremely taxing on all body systems. I believe that the stress that is generated by this constant up and down (this overstimulation/exhaustion) is one of the major factors contributing to premature aging and disease.

ALLERGIC FATIGUE AND HEREDITY As among allergic-headache sufferers, there is generally a personal or family history of allergies among tension-fatigue syndrome sufferers as well. Most of them are eventually labeled neurotic. The tendency of orthodox physicians to assume that psychosomatic disease is responsible for the syndrome stigmatizes many sufferers with a diagnosis of mental illness and leaves them to cope with their disabling symptoms alone.

DIAGNOSIS Like allergic headaches, allergic fatigue cannot be diagnosed definitely until a complete check-up rules out other factors. This check-up includes a comprehensive case history, a complete physical examination, and diagnostic allergy testing.

Other causes of nervous fatigue are chronic infections, diabetes, hypoglycemia, an inactive thyroid gland, nervous system disorders, heart disease, anemia, malignancy, and various nutrient deficiencies.

If this is a concern of yours, be sure your doctor is at least *open* to the possibility that allergy could be the culprit. Both of you should also be well aware that the diagnosis of one disease does not rule out the simultaneous presence of allergic fatigue. In such cases one can determine the degree to which the allergic fatigue is causing symptoms only after following the appropriate allergy-control program.

There are characteristic signals that support the diagnosis of allergic fatigue. As a rule, sufferers do not respond to extended vacations or rest periods, and they fail to be relieved by thyroid, estrogen, or vitamin therapy. Yet their response to allergen elimination is striking. If, despite the disappearance of other symptoms, the fatigue and weakness persist, it's possible that the allergy has been only partially corrected or that a nonallergic abnormality is also affecting the patient.

People commonly binge on foods to which they are sensitive over the weekend. This destructive habit is often responsible for the Monday morning "blahs." If you feel blue by your coffee break on Monday, sit down and examine what you have been eating during the previous few days.

Clinical ecologists suggest that elimination diets be used with all patients complaining of fatigue when no other cause is obvious.

IS YOUR CHILD SUFFERING FROM ALLERGIC FATIGUE? Children suffering from the tension-fatigue syndrome may well exhibit "opposing" symptoms. That is, they may suffer on the one hand from drowsiness, inability to concentrate, sullenness, depression, listlessness, fatigue, and poor coordination; and on the other hand from temper tantrums, belligerence, restlessness, and irritability. Mood swings are typical.

Leg aches, backaches, bed-wetting, increased salivation, and excessive sweating are other symptoms more common in infants and young children than in adults. Pediatricians have nicknamed youngsters experiencing excessive perspiring during their sleep "wet sleepers."

These allergic spells often begin with facial signs such as pallor, puffiness, and watery eyes, fixed expressions, and dark circles under the eyes. Parents notice that the children are suddenly more irritable, restless, and moody, or else listless and sleepy, for no apparent reason.

The symptoms may persist for several hours or even several days, and they may accompany another allergic reaction. For some children, this syndrome is experienced by itself, but it is more frequently accompanied by other allergic conditions, such as asthma, headache, eczema, or diarrhea.

The childhood symptoms fall into three categories: chronic fatigue and depression; hyperactivity and insomnia; and both tension and fatigue during the same episode or on different occasions. Generally, children in all three categories show signs of irritability (after all, they don't feel good), and they tend to be socially maladjusted.

A young children's allergic symptoms will appear to "evolve" as they age. Up to age three, restlessness and insomnia are the major complaints; then hyperactivity becomes the outstanding characteristic. Such children are easily upset and have frequent temper tantrums and crying spells. They appear spoiled. They may also seem dazed and unable to think clearly. When the allergy causing this behavior is treated, it is as if a fog lifts, and the child's IQ appears to increase rapidly. Because these children are high-strung and unruly, they are often difficult for parents and teachers to manage. But it is usually the symptoms of fatigue that most alarms parents. When they see their child chronically lethargic, they seek a medical opinion.

This condition often runs in families. Pediatricians remark that it's not uncommon for parents with tired and irritable children to have similar symptoms themselves.

THE JEKYLL-HYDE EFFECT Some allergic children exhibit severe psychological and nervous symptoms such as facial tics, "pins and needles," and extreme personality disturbances (including psychotic behavior). They may exhibit drastic personality changes, a Jekyll-Hyde effect, after allergen exposure. If the exposure is continuous, as when a food allergen is consumed regularly, the child may display chronic antisocial behavior. Pediatricians and parents report that these children cannot get along with their peers, often behave in a cruel and disorderly manner, and are constantly in trouble, both at home and at school.

THE PRICE OF MISDIAGNOSIS Typically, failure to properly diagnose the tension-fatigue syndrome leads to unjustifiable diagnoses and treatments. The medical literature cites numerous unnecessary operations involving tonsils, sinuses, appendices, gall bladders, and pelvic organs.

Mistaken diagnoses have included cerebral palsy, mental retardation, epilepsy, malnutrition, low protein intake, and anemia. Or barring any physiological diagnosis, the child is all too often labeled as stupid, a troublemaker, or a social misfit. The tragedy of such misdiagnoses cannot be overstated.

If left undetected, the primary allergy disorder may even result in permanent emotional problems. "It is not hard to imagine," states Dr. Frazier, "what being constantly scolded in school and at home can do to the child's self-esteem and confidence."[28]

When parents and teachers learn to understand the child's physical and mental condition through proper medical diagnosis, their attitudes usually change. They realize that the child they had labeled as bad and unruly was, in fact, sick.

DOCTORS SHOULD LISTEN TO THEIR PATIENTS One point stressed by Dr. Rowe and other early allergists more than thirty years ago is the importance of doctors paying attention to what the patient says. Unfortunately, what a patient says is often as ignored now as it was thirty years ago, when Dr. Rowe so wisely wrote, "More attention should be paid to the patient's own statements regarding his food idiosyncrasies and, above all, to a realization that food allergy is an entity."[29]

Obviously, not all disorders have their roots in allergies: therefore, a diet change is not always effective. Yet our diets are responsible for more physical and emotional ill health than most doctors and the public realize.

If only a small proportion of those affected by the tension-fatigue syndrome were relieved of their symptoms, what a wonderful impact it could have on our society! On an individual level, the gift of energy and tranquillity amounts to nothing less than a miraculous new lease on life.

OBESITY AND ALLERGY

More than 40 million people in this country today suffer from obesity. Losing weight has become a national obsession, often starting in the early teens and continuing throughout life. I know some people who have been on diets ever since I met them many years ago. Every six months or so a new national best-seller appears on the bookshelves claiming to offer a new, better, and less painful way to lose weight quickly.

It is commonly believed that people who are overweight or obese come from families that tend toward obesity, that they have a thyroid or metabolic problem, or that they just plain lack the self-discipline to curb their eating. Although these may be contributing factors, in some cases a hidden food allergy may also play a role in how much you eat. Clinical ecologists have found that in many instances, when a food allergen is eliminated from a person's diet, a welcome side effect occurs: they lose weight. On the other hand, obesity can exacerbate any allergies that you may have.

HOW ALLERGY CAN TRIGGER OBESITY Allergy may play a role in causing you to gain weight through the following mechanisms.

1. An addictive allergy causes you to crave the food to which you are allergic. This may show up simply as a craving, or you may be conditioned to consume because it relieves your withdrawal symptoms. Many of the foods to which people are commonly addicted are also high in calories: chocolate, cheese, and sugar. People gain weight by eating these high-caloric foods in response to their addictive urges. In the extreme, they may binge on an allergen, unable to stop eating it even though they are no longer hungry. This compulsive eating may be nothing more than an attempt to stave off withdrawal symptoms. It is possible in certain cases that hunger or thirst are themselves withdrawal symptoms from a given allergen, so that when a person starts to withdraw from that food or chemical, he or she feels a general need to eat or drink.

Dr. Randolph writes of one overweight patient who felt compelled to eat enormous quantities of peanut butter and bread products. The woman compared her desire to eat these foods to an alcoholic's desire to drink. Dr. Randolph tested her for food sensitivity and found that she was allergic to peanuts, yeast, and milk. When he placed the patient on a rotation diet that eliminated these foods, the woman's weight stabilized at a normal level.[30]

2. Allergies can also interfere with the body's natural ability to regulate metabolism. Human beings usually maintain their proper weight by eating the amount of food they need to function properly. When the body needs food, it sends out a hunger signal, and the individual knows it's time to eat. However, if this mechanism breaks down, the individual may get hungry even though no food is needed. Within the hypothalamus, a regulatory center of the brain, is located the appestat, which controls the conscious feeling of fullness. Allergies may temporarily impair the reactions of the appestat so that the individual continues to eat though already full.

3. Allergies can be responsible for edema, or swelling, in the feet, hands, stomach, face, or throughout the body. Many people refer to this in lay terms as "water retention" or "bloating." When it affects the whole body, it can be perceived as excess fat when it is only a build-up of liquid due to an allergic reaction.

Eating food allergens can cause fluid retention equal to as much as 4 percent of one's total body weight. Thus, from swelling alone, a 150-pound person could gain six pounds.

If you've ever lost more than three and a half pounds per week on a reducing diet—only drinking water—swelling may be a factor in your weight problem.

This greater-than-normal weight loss often occurs when an allergic individual goes on a typical reducing diet, especially if that diet eliminates food allergens. If you are sensitive to sugar, for example, and your diet restricts desserts, you will lose weight beyond what you lose from calorie restriction alone.

Allergic edema may also explain why some individuals can diet and *not* lose much weight. Some allergen still in the diet may cause fluid retention.

Chemical sensitivity may also cause edema. Take Cindy, for example. Cindy continued gaining weight despite following a low-calorie diet and a daily exercise program. Her diet, although low in calories, was high in chemical content. To cut calories, she ate lots of diet foods containing saccharine and artificial colors, flavors, and preservatives. When Cindy eliminated those chemicals from her diet, she began to lose weight, even though she was actually eating more food.

ORTHODOX TREATMENTS AND ENVIRONMENTAL ALTER-NATIVES Most people who want or need to lose weight go on some sort of a calorie-restricted diet. Over the past twenty years there have been no shortage of "miracle diets," each claiming to be better than the one before at getting you to lose weight. Judging by the number of obese people in this nation, it appears that these diets may not be working as well as they claim.

One of the reasons why these diets may not work is that they do not eliminate foods to which you are allergic. This can create all sorts of havoc. First, even if you adhere to the diet, you may still have bloating, indigestion, and metabolic irregularities. Then, once you are off the diet your withdrawal symptoms from limited intake of the allergen may cause you to binge as described above. Or you may find it almost intolerable to stay on the diet because of the limited-calorie intake coupled with the hunger sensations that are symptomatic of your allergies. It is not uncommon for people on limited-calorie diets to quickly gain back any weight they may have lost on a diet and more.

Since these diets are usually an ordeal and are often ineffective, doctors often prescribe diuretics to control water retention. These give dieters the impression that they are losing fat when in fact they are just being artificially stimulated to release water. Diuretics do nothing to get at the cause of any swelling or water retention you may have. However, they may cause potassium deficiencies, which first show up as fatigue and muscle weakness. Severe deficiencies may cause serious damage to blood, kidneys, nerves, muscles, and skin.

If you are having trouble dieting, appetite suppressants may also be prescribed. Although these may effectively suppress the appetite, helping some to lose weight, they do nothing to treat the root cause of overeating. These suppressants usually contain amphetamines, which stimulate the nervous system. They may also contain phenylpropanol-amine, which can cause nausea, headaches, nervousness, elevated blood sugar levels, insomnia, and rapid heartbeat.

Clinical ecologists approach weight loss in a different way. First, a clinical ecologist will suggest following a well-balanced diet that emphasizes whole foods and eliminates common allergens. They determine which foods and chemicals, if any, are causing the patient's problems, then design a rotation diet to prevent the development of further sensitivities, even after satisfactory weight loss has been achieved.

Exercise is an important element of a comprehensive weight-loss program. It increases the blood flow, brings needed nutrients to the cells, and encourages the elimination of toxins. As we grow older, our metabolism slows down, causing us to digest our food less rapidly and efficiently. Exercise, which causes an increase in metabolic rate, can counteract this slowdown. This is more than just the simple burning of calories. We all know that we burn more calories when we run than when we sit. The change in metabolic rate that I am talking about is a constant change. Hence, exercise itself not only causes calories to be burned while you exercise, it also causes your metabolic rate to increase, such that you burn more calories than you ordinarily would even when you are not exercising. After a good physical exercise, you will feel a good kind of "tired," a relaxed "tired" that is the natural response to exertion. This will bring you to relax more easily.

Many people say that exercise makes them ravenous. My response to this is that they probably did not exercise strenuously enough. I have often been hungry going into a workout, but have not wanted to eat beforehand because it would make me feel heavy. At first, when I start to exercise, I am still hungry; then about ten minutes into the workout, it goes away. It's not that I have forgotten it; the hunger is just not there. Then an hour or so after the exercise, I feel it come back. By this time I am relaxed, and at the same time I feel good about myself and my body. I am not about to eat nervously (which often leads to a binge), as I would have done before the exercise. Physical exertion increases blood flow, bringing needed nutrients to the cells, and it tends to calm the mood, breaking down one's nervous habits.

Alan Levin, M.D., suggests that overweight patients follow a special diet that checks for obesity-related allergies. This diet eliminates salt, sugar, and tap water. Simultaneously, over a period of five weeks, the individual tests for a common allergen such as milk, wheat, corn, eggs, chocolate, or yeast. Each of these foods is avoided for four days. If, after that period, the individual has lost five or more pounds, the test food is labeled a potential allergen and is avoided for at least two months. Then the individual reintroduces it on a rotational basis, checking to make sure that it is no longer causing problems.[31]

Dr. Marshall Mandell, a leading clinical ecologist who practices in Norwalk, Connecticut, and is the coauthor of *Dr. Mandell's 5-Day Allergy Relief System*, recommends that when following a rotation diet, patients should weigh themselves daily to check for water retention. He also points out that after the withdrawal period a rotation diet and avoiding allergens can help halt food cravings, thus interrupting compulsive eating patterns.[32]

ARTHRITIS AND ALLERGY

TWO TYPES OF ARTHRITIS   More than 25 million Americans, including 250,000 children, suffer from arthritis. It is a painful, unpredictable, and crippling disease that the medical establishment, for the most part, considers incurable. The word *arthritis* means "inflammation of the joints." The disease seems to affect different people in different ways. It can affect a single joint, or it can spread to every joint of the body; it can leave the victim in constant pain, or it can flare up and subside. Sometimes it disappears for good on its own.

There are two basic types of arthritis. The first, *osteoarthritis*, often occurs in joints that have been stressed through injury, repeated exertion, or overuse, as in some sports. In this type the cartilage around the joint begins to wear away, causing bone to scrape bone, which produces a sort of grating sound and a stiffness in the affected joint. This type of arthritis is so common that it is often said simply to be part of the normal aging process. The frequency with which arthritis occurs, coupled with the fact that it is a disease and not a "normal" state for human beings, leads me to suspect that often what we may unquestioningly accept as our fate may in fact be preventable, and that the normal aging process, in which *normal* is taken to mean "free of disease," does not necessarily include the stiffening that is so commonly associated with old age.

The second type is *rheumatoid arthritis*, which is the more serious and also the more erratic of the two. It primarily strikes women between the ages of twenty and forty. Here the arthritis causes the cartilage to be eaten away. Scar tissue forms, and bones may actually fuse together, resulting in severe pain and restriction in movement. Strange as it may seem, this form of arthritis particularly is subject to flareups, followed by remissions. Ten to 20 percent of rheumatoid arthritis actually disappears by itself and does not reappear.

THE TRADITIONAL APPROACH   Arthritis is yet another condition that baffles the medical establishment. It is called incurable and is most commonly treated with aspirin. Even though we are told that research is being done to find a cure, after years of unfruitful efforts and millions of dollars spent the Arthritis Foundation and other entities conducting this research still do not appear to be close to a cure.

Americans currently spend in excess of $2 billion annually on arthritis drugs. Aspirin is the biggest seller, and because it is an over-the-counter drug, most people erroneously assume that it is safe. But any drug taken over a long period of time, especially in the quantities that arthritis sufferers require to relieve their pain, can and does present health problems. One of the most common problems with aspirin is that it eats away at the stomach lining, which protects it from digestive juices. The result is bleeding ulcers that can bleed for up to two days. People like arthritis sufferers who take aspirin daily have a much greater chance of contracting this stomach bleeding. Aspirin can also cause burning in the esophagus, the tube that runs from your mouth to your stomach.

Aspirin has also been reported to cause kidney failure. One study revealed that 20 percent of its cases of kidney failure were due to aspirin. Another study reported that the long-acting aspirin now promoted for arthritis caused 28 percent of users to go deaf, compared to less than one percent of patients taking regular aspirin.

Acetaminophen was developed to get around many of the problems caused by aspirin. But it is just as toxic and causes extensive damage to the liver. Both aspirin and acetaminophen destroy vitamins A and C, which play a major role in reducing stress. These vitamins are of particular importance to the arthritis sufferer, in whom stress often triggers arthritis attacks. Vitamin C is also responsible for building up the connective tissue, collagen. Collagen destruction by large doses of aspirin may further the deterioration of the cartilage in arthritis.

Physicians frequently prescribe steroids in the treatment of arthritis. The most commonly used steroid is cortisone. Cortisone is a synthetic adrenal hormone that reduces inflammation. It is a powerful anti-inflammatory, but it also has very serious side effects.

Inflammation is part of the body's natural healing mechanism. When a wound gets red and itches, that means the body is healing it. For some time now it has been noticed that cortisone interferes with the healing of wounds, probably because it shuts off the inflammation stage. Instead of going through the natural healing process, wounds remain at an intermediate stage of healing, often in the form of open sores. Cortisone has also been known to interfere with the body's formation of collagen. It is responsible for stunted growth in children and depression, and it causes the adrenals to malfunction and eventually atrophy with prolonged use. Recently, cortisone has been linked to prostate cancer.

When a steroid is injected into a specific site, there is less chance of an adverse reaction because the drug does not circulate through the entire body. But an injected dose is not as effective as an oral dose.

If injections do provide pain relief, it is usually short-lived.

Many physicians still prescribe another group of drugs known as nonsteroidal antiinflammatory drugs. These drugs, such as Napricin and Motrin, have fewer side effects than do steroids, but they are also less effective. Dr. Mandell points out that these medications may offer little more relief than aspirin and are a good deal more expensive.[33]

Several other commonly used arthritis treatments, too, have side effects. Gold injections, for example, may cause skin rashes, inflammation of the kidneys, and changes in bone marrow.

Occasionally, doctors may even administer anticancer drugs, but these are highly toxic and may in fact be cancer-causing in the long run.

These drugs may be effective at relieving the pain of arthritis, but none of them treats its cause.

GOING TO THE HEART OF THE PROBLEM   It appears to this author that the general concensus among orthodox physicians is that arthritis is a mysterious disease for which there is no known cure or treatment, only drugs to relieve the pain. However, many clinical ecologists challenge this consensus for a variety of reasons.

First, clinical ecologists ask, is it mere coincidence that arthritis often follows the pattern of allergic reactions. For instance, swelling and inflammation (e.g., hives, puffiness under eyes) which frequently accompany allergy. It seems likely that arthritis, which by definition is an inflammation of the joints, may in some cases at least be attributable to allergy. Also, the erratic nature of arthritis is noticeably similar to that of many food allergies; it flares up and goes away by itself, or it remains constant. In a cyclic allergy, which clinical ecologists have found constitute the vast majority of all allergies, symptoms flare up after a food allergen has been eaten and subside once the food is eliminated from the system. If the food is eaten on a regular basis, the symptoms may be chronic and never let up.

Although traditional practitioners are not willing to admit a relationship between allergy and arthritis in general, some of them do acknowledge that elimination of foods from the nightshade family seems to help in some cases of arthritis. This was first discovered by Norman Childers, Ph.D., a horticulturalist at Rutgers University. He had read that cattle exhibited arthritic symptoms after grazing on plants in this family. Dr. Childers decided to eliminate foods of the nightshade family—namely potatoes, tomatoes, peppers and eggplants—in an attempt to relieve his own arthritis. He found that this worked. After meeting resistance and skepticism from the medical establishment, Dr. Childers enlisted a number of people across the country to try eliminating the nightshades. A majority reported partial relief when these foods were eliminated from their diets.[34] It is thought that one reason for the relief is some arthritics' sensitivity to solanine, a substance found in potatoes that is highly toxic. The average American consumes up to 9,700 milligrams of solanine per year, a dose large enough to literally kill a horse. For those who eat potatoes regularly, this substance may never be fully eliminated, resulting in an arthritislike allergic reaction.

Those traditional practitioners who did acknowledge the correlation between the nightshades and arthritis usually stopped there. Clinical ecologists, however, used Dr. Childers's work as a springboard. If sensitivity to nightshades could trigger arthritic flareups, the ecologists hypothesized, then maybe other sorts of sensitivities were involved in arthritis, too. Dr. Marshall Mandell believes that 80 to 90 percent of all arthritis cases may in fact be due to allergies. This "pseudo-arthritis" will in most cases be diagnosed and treated as arthritis. It may actually develop into a full-blown case of arthritis if not treated properly. But at least at the beginning it may be just your body's way of manifesting an allergy to a given food or chemical. Accordingly, clinical ecologists believe that examining "arthritic" patients for food allergies is essential. It can reduce current symptoms, prevent new ones, and minimize the damage that can result from continual joint inflammation.

The link between arthritis and allergy is still not widely accepted, but the concept is not new. As early as 1917 it was suggested that there might be a relationship between food allergies and arthritis in some patients.

In 1949, Michael Zeller, M.D., an allergist who practiced in Chicago, published a study of patients whose rheumatoid arthritis cleared up after they avoided food allergens. One patient was a forty-one-year-old woman who had had pain and swelling in her wrist and finger joints for five years. Swelling had also developed in her knees and shoulders. She was in constant pain; changes in the weather worsened her symptoms. The woman also had symptoms commonly seen in allergic individuals, such as sneezing attacks, stuffy nose, abdominal distention, stomach cramps, and almost-daily episodes of diarrhea.

Dr. Zeller suspected that allergy might be playing a role in her arthritic symptoms. When he tested her, he found that she was allergic to dust, pork, milk, lettuce, string beans, and potatoes. After these foods were eliminated from her diet, the severity of her arthritis was tremendously reduced.

In the 1950s, William Kaufman, M.D., Ph.D., of Stratford, Connecticut, did a study on forty-seven of his patients suffering from arthritis. This study showed a definite relationship between arthritis and allergy. Some patients reported complete relief from joint stiffness after they began to avoid foods and chemicals to which they were allergic.

Dr. Kaufman also noted that the difference in symptoms that arthritis sufferers exhibit. He suggested that the reason why some people suffer constant pain is because they are in constant contact with the allergen causing their arthritis; that is, they eat the food on a regular basis, and their bodies are never totally free of it. Intermittent pain, on the other hand, came from eating a food that they only ate occasionally.

The resemblance of arthritic symptoms to many allergic responses is almost too obvious to be ignored. I referred to the inflammation and cyclic nature of the two conditions earlier. Similarly, just as most food allergy symptoms clear up after fasting, clinical ecologists have observed that in many cases the same holds true for arthritic symptoms. They abate after fasting and reappear when normal diets are resumed. It has been noted that arthritis sufferers react most frequently to corn, wheat, and meat.

As for other food allergies, there is no one food that specifically causes arthritic symptoms. Often the foods that a person eats the most are the cause, but this is not always the case. If you suffer from arthritis, you may want to experiment with your diet and take a close look at your environment before you start taking drugs to relieve the pain. The pain may be telling you something that you need to know. Notice, for example, when your arthritis flares up, if it is cyclical; if it is constant, there may be times when it is worse than others. See if you can find a correlation between something that you ate, drank, inhaled, or touched and your arthritic pain. If you find one, try eliminating it for a week or two. It costs nothing, and it may dramatically improve your well-being.

VITAMIN AND MINERAL SUPPLEMENTS AND EXERCISE   Clinical ecologists consider other factors when treating a patient for arthritis. One of the most important is adequate calcium intake. In arthritis, calcium deposits are often found around the joints. Contrary to what you might expect, this is due not to too much calcium but to a calcium deficiency. When you lack calcium, your body draws calcium from the bones. It often draws too much. The excess calcium is then deposited at various sites in the body, especially around the joints, which can aggravate the inflammation and the stiffness of your arthritis. Thus a good physician will always check calcium intake. Since calcium deficiency may be due to a digestive malfunction, he or she will also check to make sure that you are properly absorbing the calcium you do take in. Your physician may also prescribe vitamins C and D since they can aid in calcium absorption.

If you use cortisone or antiinflammatory drugs, you should make sure to take several grams extra of vitamin C to minimize the damage done by these drugs (especially with respect to collagen formation). You may also want to supplement your diet with other immune and stress-reducing nutrients such as vitamin A, B complex, E, zinc, selenium, and magnesium, since immune malfunction and stress may also play a role in your outbreaks of joint pain.

The right type and amount of exercise are also important to retard stiffness and improve circulation. Some physicians believe that an accumulation of toxins around a joint promotes inflammation. Exercises such as swimming, t'ai chi, and yoga allow the affected joints to move without the stress that could cause injury, and they improve circulation, which aids in the elimination of toxins from the blood.

CHAPTER FOUR

Treatments

UNDERSTANDING ALLERGY

Clinical ecologists recognize that a great many more reactions are allergic than do traditional allergists, who recognize only IgE- and other immune-mediated reactions as allergic. To clinical ecologists these sensitivities constitute a mere 5 percent of all allergies. Moreover, traditional allergists usually offer only two types of treatment – namely, allergen avoidance and immunotherapy (allergy shots); whereas clinical ecologists' treatments are much more comprehensive. For example, clinical ecologists will not just tell you to avoid a given allergen; they will also give you a rotational diet so that you do not develop any new food allergies. Clinical ecologists will also check your digestive system, which may be playing a role in your allergies. They will give you vitamins, minerals, and a diet to bolster the immune system and help it function more effectively. Neutralization therapy will be used to control your symptoms, should you be exposed to the allergies.

IMMUNOTHERAPY VERSUS NEUTRALIZATION THERAPY

Immunotherapy is the primary aggressive treatment of the traditional allergists. Basically, in immunotherapy the physician administers gradual increments of a patient's allergen until the symptoms are blocked. That amount is called *optimal dose*. The concept behind it is that the patient will "use up" all of his or her antibodies to fight the shot and then will develop a higher tolerance to the substance. Immunotherapy does work for some IgE-mediated allergies, especially hay fever and pollen-related allergies. It is not, however, very effective for fighting food, animal dander, and dust allergies. It is also time-consuming and requires frequent visits to the doctor, and generally no noticeable effects are achieved until the optimal dose is achieved.

The clinical ecologist's alternative to immunotherapy is the neutralizing dose, which is effective in eight out of ten cases of patients allergic to such things as foods, chemicals, perfumes, and cigarette smoke.

In practice, neutralization therapy is exactly the opposite of immunotherapy. In immunotherapy, gradual *increments* are made in the allergen until the patient gets used to or builds up an immunity to the allergen. Because this is an adaptive process, it can take up to six months for the person to build up sufficient resistance to the allergen to be able to tolerate real-world exposure to it. By contrast, the neutralizing dose is arrived at by gradually *diluting* the allergen. The neutralizing dose is the dilution that relieves or "neutralizes" the patient's symptoms. If you are confused by this, don't worry; you are not alone. One of the major arguments that orthodox medicine makes against clinical ecology is that neutralization therapy makes no sense, that it cannot be explained scientifically, and that thus it is unproven and a sham. Yet it does work – clinical ecologists have videotapes and clinical cases to prove it.

One of the advantages of neutralization therapy over immunotherapy is that because the neutralizing dose decreases rather than increases, the quantity of the allergen can be determined in one or two sessions rather than in the six months needed for the body to adapt to immunotherapy. It also works in a much wider variety of cases than does immunotherapy. Neutralization therapy can be administered by injection or sublingually. (The latter is obviously preferred by children.) Additionally, patients can take the drops home to administer their own treatments, thus saving the time and expense of multiple visits to the doctor's office.

ROTATION DIET
. . . .

One of the most significant discoveries by clinical ecologists is that 95 percent of all allergies are cyclic rather than fixed. This means that most people are not allergic per se but rather develop allergies by over-consuming a given good.

The rotational diet was developed to address this problem in two ways. First, if you have mild sensitivities, you may be able to continue to eat the food to which you are sensitive, but only after a thorough elimination diet and then no more often than once every four days. Second, the rotational diet keeps you from developing new allergies.

It is important to fully understand the mechanism of this diet so to repeat what was said earlier, here's how the diet could work. Suppose you have a mild allergy to wheat. You go on an elimination diet, and your doctor decides to see how you feel if you eat wheat on a rotational basis. Since you like cereal in the morning, on day one you eat oatmeal, on day two puffed rice, on day three cornflakes, and on day four wheat or bran cereal. For lunch you may like sandwiches. But if you ate your wheat for breakfast, you cannot have a sandwich on wheat bread. So you may decide with your doctor to substitute a millet or barley cereal for the wheat cereal in the morning.

Sandwiches may require some flexibility unless you can find breads that are made from different grains but do not contain wheat. However, be careful not to start "abusing" other grains. Your doctor may recommend that you have fruit salad with cheese for lunch on day one; soup and salad on day two; a sandwich on the third day (this could be your wheat splurge); and a different kind of soup with salad on day four.

For dinner, if you are a meat eater, you might have beef on day one, chicken on day two, fish on day three, and lamb on day four. Remember that these should be roasted, grilled, or baked and not breaded, since you are avoiding wheat. You should also rotate the grains or vegetables you eat with the meat, although most people can eat salad greens (lettuce, watercress, parsley) and green vegetables more frequently than other foods without developing sensitivities. It's all individual; you will have to work with your physician to design the diet that is right for you. That diet will focus on eliminating the foods that contribute to your allergies in a way that is comfortable enough for you to easily work into your life. For those who are highly susceptible to new sensitivities, a five-, seven-, or even twelve-day cycle may be necessary.

The purpose of the rotational diet is to ensure not only that patients avoid their allergens but also that they do not develop new sensitivities. What often happens if patients do not follow a rotational diet is that by substituting for the eliminated food, they begin to eat foods formerly eaten infrequently and then become sensitive to those foods. Clinical ecologists recognize that an individual who is allergic to one food is susceptible to developing allergies to other foods as well; one particular allergy is not an isolated health problem.

After patients have followed a rotational diet for six weeks to six months, depending on the case, the physician may retest their sensitivity to some of the eliminated foods. Those foods to which the patient is no longer sensitive may be added to the diet on a rotational basis.

I'll discuss the details of establishing an allergy-free diet in Chapter 7.

BOOSTING THE IMMUNE SYSTEM

Our immune systems protect us from a constant onslaught of invaders that, if unchecked, could easily spell our demise. Acquired Immune Deficiency Syndrome (AIDS) is an example of what happens when our immune system shuts down and is no longer capable of defending us. When this occurs, we become prey to virtually every disease known and have no weapons with which to fight them. AIDS shows us that without a healthy immune system, the precarious balance between life and death swings toward death.

If our immune system is healthy, our resistance is high and we resist disease and interact with our environment from a position of strength. On the other hand, if our immune system is weak, the result can be AIDS, cancer, bacterial, viral, or fungal infections, arthritis, and of course allergies.

The immune system is strong and tenacious, but it has to work hard to maintain our health and it needs all the help it can get. Any number of things, either alone or in concert, can lower our immunity. Among the most common are:

- Stress
- Environmental chemicals
- Candida albicans
- Disease
- Poor nutrition and dietary habits
- Free radicals

Once the immune system succumbs to any of these factors, it may go on a downward spiral. For example, in his outstanding book *The Yeast Connection*, William G. Crook, M.D., discusses the relationship between candida albicans and allergies. Candida albicans are fungi (yeast) normally present in the mouth, digestive tract, and vagina. They are normally kept in check by our intestinal flora and other beneficial bacteria. However, when we take antibiotics, they kill not only the harmful bacteria but also the helpful bacteria that control the candida fungi. The result is that the fungi begin to multiply, rapidly causing toxins to be released into the body that weaken the immune system. When this occurs the poisoned immune system begins to malfunction, and allergies can be the result.[1]

All factors that weaken the immune system pave the way for it to malfunction at a later date. Candida albicans can contribute to allergies, as do stress and infection. Environmental pollution may cause allergies that in turn weaken the immune system and make it unable to defend against infection or cancer.

Conversely, boosting the immune system can have an overall beneficial effect on our well-being. In general, to increase your resistance to allergies or to any other disorder, you must establish a healthy routine involving:

- a nutritious diet with supplementation
- an appropriate exercise program
- stress management
- ample rest

ESSENTIAL NUTRIENTS

A number of nutrients act to strengthen the immune system. Many of them operate to neutralize free radicals, which are a major drain on our resistance. Among these are vitamins A (in the form of beta carotene, a vitamin A precursor), C, and E; the amino acid L-glutathione; and the minerals manganese, selenium, and zinc.

A free radical is a molecule that has a free electron in its outer shell, making it highly reactive. Free radicals arise from any number of sources, including ultraviolet and X-rays, yeasts, alcohol, toxic metals such as aluminum in cookware and cadmium or lead in paints, tobacco smoke, stress, illness, constipation, and free radicals themselves. Certain nutrients limit the damage done by donating an electron that "clinches" (deactivates) it. If it is not "clinched" by a free radical scavenger such as the above nutrients, the free radical can link up with anything in sight. This often causes a chain reaction, linking and combining molecules that have no business being together. The end result is cell damage and disease. The loss of elasticity in the skin as it ages is the result of free radicals that cause collagen molecules to improperly link together. By reacting with lubricants in the joints or with collagen in the connective tissues of tendons and ligaments, they can decrease joint lubrication and flexibility, causing arthritis or arthritislike symptoms.

The foremost free radical scavenger is vitamin C. In times of stress, infection, fatigue, or allergic reaction, excessive free radicals are released, thus increasing the need for vitamin C. Robert Cathcart, M.D., a physician practicing in Los Altos, California, uses megadoses of vitamin C to treat AIDS patients. He refers to vitamin C as providing "spoonfuls of electrons" that "clinch" the free radicals and render them harmless. According to Dr. Cathcart, AIDS patients are able to take and use up to 50 grams of vitamin C per day to "clinch" the free radicals that are released in their bodies due to massive infection.

Vitamin E, another potent free radical scavenger, is especially effective in intercepting the free radicals released by rancid fats and unsaturated fats, such as most vegetable oils, which rapidly *oxidize* (become transformed into free radicals) when exposed to oxygen. They are one of the largest sources of free radicals in our diets. It is now thought that vitamin E's sole purpose may be to act as an *antioxidant* by donating electrons to these oxidized fats, thus preventing them from causing damage. Because all unsaturated fats oxidize rapidly (with the exception of linseed and olive oils, which contain natural antioxidants), some people recommend using saturated fats like butter to replace oils in cooking. However, this can raise problems for people on restricted cholesterol diets or who have allergies to dairy. The sensible solution is to make sure that you take ample amounts of vitamin E and lower your fat and oil consumption in general. (I will say more about fats in Chapter 7.)

All the nutrients listed at the beginning of this section are equally important, as they each play a specific role in fighting to limit the damage done by free radicals. Vitamins C and E are called general or nonspecific free radical scavengers.

Other nutrients that have been found to strengthen and stimulate the immune system are B complex; the amino acids L-cysteine and L-arginine; the minerals magnesium, iron, and copper; and chlorophyll and garlic.

While each of the components of the B complex has a specific role, the complex is generally used to reduce stress, which is a major immune depletor. Both riboflavin (vitamin B_2) and niacin (vitamin B_3) are required for certain enzymes in the body's normal free radical neutralization process. This renders these toxic ions into harmless agents. Thiamine (vitamin B_1) is responsible for ensuring that our bodies produce energy efficiently and effectively. Without this steady flow of energy, we become tired and depressed, and our immune system has a hard time doing the work its supposed to do. Pantothenic Acid (vitamin B_5) also helps convert our foods into energy and helps manufacture antibodies to fight infections in the body. A deficiency of pyridoxine (vitamin B_6), which requires magnesium as a cofactor, has been shown to cause mental and nervous disorders. The body requires it to manufacture lecithin, a natural fatty acid that works to dissolve cholestrol deposits in the arteries. Accordingly, vitamin B_6 plays an important role in reducing the risks of athero scelerosis and heart disease. Abram Hoffer, M.D., an esteemed Canadian physician who has done extensive research on the effects of vitamins in treating mental disorders, has found that vitamin B_6 is especially effective in treating hyperactivity in children. Dr. Hoffer reported in his book *Mental and Elemental Nutrients* that he did studies showing that many schizophrenic patients improve dramatically when given megadoses of niacin (vitamin B_3).

Garlic and chlorophyll work as blood purifiers, stimulate circulation, and strengthen our resistance. Both these substances are also effective fungicides and therefore help to prevent candida albicans, which, as I mentioned earlier, can be a major drain on the immune system.

STRESS REDUCTION

In addition to dietary changes, other factors are also important for attaining optimal health and well-being. One is stress reduction.

In previous chapters I have explained the role that stress may play in allergies in general and in fatigue-related allergies in particular. It may tax the immune system and cause it to function improperly, or it may cause chemicals to be released to which your body reacts allergically. You should therefore find a way that works for you to reduce stress in your daily life. Stress-reducing techniques such as progressive relaxation and biofeedback essentially involve reconditioning the body to learn a new way to deal with stress.

In *progressive relaxation* you lie comfortably on the floor or on a bed, your arms at your sides and your feet about shoulder width apart. Tapes are available on the market that take you through the steps I will describe below, but you can also do it on your own.

Once in this position, start at your toes. Relax them completely. Feel all the tension going out of them. Move to your feet and ankles and progressively up your body doing the same thing. Relax and feel the tension go out; let the weight of your body go into the floor. Don't forget any part of your body. Concentrate on areas such as shoulders, neck, and forehead that are especially apt to hold the day's tension.

There are many variations on the technique of progressive relaxation. Once you are physically relaxed, you may want to try to equally relax your mind by letting all thoughts flow out of it and remaining totally silent for an additional fifteen minutes to half hour. Or you may want to put on some especially soothing music while you are relaxing. Then let your mind flow with the music once you are relaxed. You may also use visualization techniques, in which you create in your mind a beautiful environment, say a beach in Tahiti, a country house next to a lake, or a lovely garden. Then, once you are relaxed, you go to this place to rejuvenate yourself.

Whatever technique you use, you should always do your relaxations at a time when you will not be disturbed. Take the phone off the hook, close the door to your room, and tell others in the house that you need a half hour to yourself.

Progressive relaxation is often used in conjunction with self-hypnosis, in which you first put yourself into a state of total relaxation and then use certain positive affirmations to encourage behavioral change. Complete relaxation is the trancelike state that hypnotists induce; you become open to suggestions. If you have trouble with allergies, you may want to suggest something to yourself like, "My immune system is getting stronger. It's able to distinguish grass pollen from harmful bacteria." Or if you have trouble with overeating and obesity, you might want to tell yourself that you love your body, and that from now on you will only eat foods that promote its beauty and slimness.

Visualization is another technique that can be used to enhance your overall well-being. Drs. Carl and Stephanie Simonton, pioneers of visualization for the treatment of disease, have had much success in using this technique with cancer patients. You try to create a specific visual image like the beach in Tahiti, but this time the image is of you being happy and healthy. You can actually create a visual image of your antibodies battling the disease or of your cells regenerating themselves.

In *biofeedback*, an electronic device is wired to your body. You listen on headphones or watch the patterns of your involuntary responses on a monitor. You learn which sounds or patterns signify relaxation, and you then learn to voluntarily produce them.

Biofeedback can be used to voluntarily relax muscles or to raise the temperature of the skin (which is often lowered in response to stress). Alan Levin, M.D., a leading preventive medicine specialist, described one patient who was aided by working with biofeedback. She was able to clear up most of her food sensitivities by dietary means but was unable to control her migraine headaches. By using biofeedback, the woman learned to raise her skin temperature. This prevented the constriction of blood vessels, which had been triggering her migraines.

OTHER WAYS TO FIGHT STRESS AND RELAX   Many other techniques, such as meditation, yoga and t'ai chi, all of which promote physical and mental relaxation, can also reduce stress.

In addition to formal techniques, any relaxing activity may be beneficial. Painting, playing a musical instrument, singing, listening to music, or spending time with a friend – any of these pastimes could take your mind off anxieties. In short, enjoy yourself!

EXERCISE: AN ALL-AROUND TONIC

The benefits of exercise cannot be overemphasized. Most people know that they should exercise, but even with the current "fitness kick," still only a very small segment of the population actually gets adequate exercise. The results are obesity, back and circulation problems, stress, weak immune systems, and disease.

When we do not exercise for long periods of time, our muscles begin to atrophy and our joints stiffen. Over time this means that our stomach muscles are no longer able to hold our organs in place; they tend to descend with the pull of gravity. The muscles in the back no longer hold our posture erect, and we become stooped and have lower back pain, which is compounded by the organs that have moved from their original position and exert pressure on the lower vertebrae. Without constant motion joints lose their mobility, and bones tend to fuse together, severely restricting movement.

Lack of exercise causes the blood to circulate more slowly. Substances are not eliminated as quickly as they should be, and they can build up in toxic amounts. The liver is overworked, digestion becomes sluggish, and constipation may occur, followed by prostate, colon, kidney, and liver diseases. Exercise also brings oxygen into the system, which helps in the digestion of food; without adequate oxygen our brains become sluggish and inattentive, and fatigue results.

When you do not exercise fat infiltrates and replaces muscle tissue. If you are a man, your body should be about 15 percent fat; if you are a woman, 22 percent. Most men have about 23 percent fat, and most women, 36 percent. This accounts for the marked difference in appearance between a runner, for example, and a typical American.

The difference is not simply the lower body weight; the lean, trim physique of the runner comes from a lower percentage of body fat as well. When you exercise, muscle replaces fat. Muscle weighs more than fat, so when you first start exercising you may actually gain some weight. Don't be alarmed; you are eliminating fat, which is what dieting is supposed to be about. After a couple weeks, if you have fat to lose, the deposits on your legs, hips, stomach, and arms will start to be burned. You may find that it was not weight that you needed to lose as much as fat.

Kenneth Cooper, M.D., an aerobic fitness specialist in Dallas, Texas, has found that some of the top athletes today – Hershall Walker, for instance – have under 2 percent body fat. On the other hand, Dr. Cooper estimates that some 60 million Americans are over their acceptable weights. He discusses the fat-versus-weight issue as follows:

> What happens in a state of inactivity or sedentary living? Many things. One is that these people tend to increase their body weight, but along with that, there is also an increase in body fat. I want to make that point clear. Because you can't just look at a person's height and weight and say that this person is overweight... just by looking at the scales. You must have some means of determining percentage of body fat, and we do this by skin-fold thickness, by underwater weighing, and by various other techniques. Because we have found that there is a relationship between *fat* and hypertension, *fat* and abnormal cholesterol, *fat* and heart disease, not weight per se. It's an important point.[2]

Without proper exercise our metabolism becomes sluggish. You may find that as you get older, you have to watch what you eat much more carefully, and even then you still seem to put on weight. With age the metabolism begins to slow down. This process can be aggravated by inadequate exercise, or it can be offset with a proper exercise program. The increased oxygen level you get from exercise results in an increased rate of metabolism, and you burn food more quickly and efficiently.

Not only does exercise help burn calories, replace muscle, displace fat, and increase your metabolic rate; it also works as a natural appetite suppressant. According to Dr. Cooper,

"Exercise helps you to control your body weight, particularly if you exercise at the end of the day, prior to the evening meal. Exercise helps to control the enormous number of calories many of us eat in the evening meal, which I think, accounts for the massive amounts of obesity in this country."[3]

To summarize, lack of exercise can lead to:

- obesity
- cardiovascular disorders
- a weakened immune system
- muscular and skeletal weakness and pain
- fatigue
- liver problems
- indigestion
- stress
- disease

Adequate exercise promotes:

- low body fat
- proper circulation
- a healthy immune system
- strength and flexibility
- efficient digestion
- energy
- relaxation
- a decrease in appetite

To obtain the maximum benefit from your exercise, I recommend some form of sustained aerobic stimulation for a minimum of twenty minutes four days a week. If you are a group-oriented person or have trouble motivating yourself, you may want to look into aerobic exercise classes. All you have to do is get yourself to the class, and if the instructor is good, he or she will take over from there. If you have a previous history of injury, heart problems, are over age forty, or have not exercised for a while, you should have a good physical examination and talk with your physician before you begin. You may also want to shop around for the class that suits you best. Exaggerated movements and a lot of jerking and pounding should be avoided; they can cause injury, especially if you start to become fatigued ten to fifteen minutes into the workout. You may also want to read books that can give you more detailed information on the proper type of aerobic exercise.

If you are self-motivated or cannot leave the house, you may want to try to work out with an exercise video. Jane Fonda's workouts are excellent and are now available in a low-impact version, in versions for pregnant women and for beginning and advanced exercisers.

Jogging and race-walking are excellent forms of aerobic exercise, but they are not for everybody. If your resistance to them can be traced to laziness, I heartily encourage you to overcome this, maybe with a friend or by joining a running group in your area. The benefits of both these forms of exercise are immeasurable; in very little time your energy level and disposition will improve, and you should have little trouble motivating yourself. One reason runners often seem hooked on running is that after fifteen to twenty minutes endorphins begin to be released by the brain. These are naturally occuring, soothing substances that cause mood elevation, a sort of natural "high" that gives the runner a pleasant, vibrant sense of well-being.

If you are advised by your physician not to jog, you may want to try race-walking, which provides all the benefits of jogging without stress on joints or impact on the body. Books are available in the health and exercise section of your local bookstore on the technique and benefits of race-walking.

You must choose the kind of exercise that is right for you. It should be something that you can do without injuring yourself and that still gives you a good workout; you should like it, which is one reason why swimming is an ideal exercise for so many people. It should be something that manageably fits into your lifestyle. This does not mean that if "it's too much trouble," don't do it. If you are not currently exercising, chances are any effort to exercise will seem like too much trouble. However, if you decide that you want to exercise at a gym, you should choose one that is either close to your home or place of work. Do not let your initial zeal and good resolutions make you take on more than you can handle by choosing a gym in an inconvenient location. Otherwise the location of the gym, not your resolve, may keep you from exercising.

You should also choose the exercise that is right for you. If you have an allergy to chlorine, for example, swimming is not the ideal exercise for you unless you live close to a lake or ocean. If you are asthmatic, you may have trouble with cold air and so should not exercise out of doors in winter.

You may also want to vary your exercise to make sure you are getting conditioned all over; most exercises tend to emphasize one group of muscles or one aspect of fitness. For example, you may jog or race-walk three days a week and do a stretching and toning exercise another day or two a week. Swimming is considered the ideal exercise in that it gives a cardiovascular workout and strengthens, tones, and firms muscles without shortening them.

A WORD ON CHIROPRACTIC THERAPY

In addition to treatments that work to strengthen the immune system, chiropractic therapy has been found to be useful for many patients who experience chronic fatigue, headaches, muscle spasms, or asthma. The theory behind chiropractic is that when vertebrae are even subtly out of place, a break in proper nerve impulse transmission results; this triggers a physiological reaction somewhere in the body. When a chiropractor realigns the vertebrae, the nervous system is restored to a state of healthy functioning.

DIGESTIVE IMBALANCE

So we have seen, digestive problems often play a role in the development of allergies. If you go to see a clinical ecologist and are found to have difficulty digesting your foods, you may be given betaine or some other natural form of hydrochloric acid to help you break down your foods more effectively. Betaine usually comes in tablet form and is available at most health-food stores. It is used to correct digestive difficulties resulting from inadequate stomach secretion of hydrochloric acid. Thorough chewing of one's food is also essential to proper digestion. There are digestive enzymes in the saliva that break down starches, and if the food is rushed down, these enzymes do not have a chance to work. Additional burden is thus placed on the intestinal enzymes.

But do not self-medicate. The problem may be either too much or too little stomach acid. If you take antacid tables when you have low stomach acid or take hydrochloric acid when you're overly acidic, you will only make the problem worse.

MINIMIZING THE POLLUTION IN OUR LIVES
. . . .

It is important for allergic patients to reduce their exposure to chemicals in order to regain their health. This is obviously necessary for the chemically sensitive, and it may also be beneficial for those with other allergies, since any exposure to chemicals taxes the immune system.

The place to start is in the home. Clinical ecologists may recommend that patients eliminate gas stoves and heaters. According to one study conducted at the University of California, the carbon monoxide and nitrogen dioxide levels even in kitchens with a properly vented gas stove were found to be equivalent to those in the Los Angeles air on a smoggy day. In kitchens with unvented stoves, the levels were three times those of Los Angeles smog. Gas stoves and heaters may also have leaks. Remember the case given by Dr. Rapp in Chapter 1, in which exposure to a gas leak led to sensitivities to other chemicals later on. Dr. Randolph also relates the case of a forty-four-year-old housewife who became almost a physical invalid because of exposure to gas. This woman had suffered from childhood from headaches, backaches, stuffy nose, motion sickness, and hyperactivity. Her problems always got worse in a gas-equipped kitchen. She frequently dropped dishes and never learned to cook because of clumsiness and irritability in the kitchen. As a child she instinctively avoided the house and spent most of her time out of doors. She was often chastised for using rouge because her cheeks were so red.

After she married, the rooms in her house were painted. After being exposed to paint fumes over a two-week period, her symptoms were aggravated. Then she developed allergies to foods and suffered constantly from colds and infections of unknown origin. She tried taking up pottery, which she had always loved, but she had to discontinue it because of fumes from the gas-fired kiln.

She lost weight and at one point was down to eighty-five pounds. Dcotors prescribed various medications, but none of them worked.

Dr. Randolph says that she acted so strangely that her husband and doctor believed that she was a drug addict. Her husband even beat her once to get her to own up to her addiction. His belief seemed to be borne out after she improved in the hospital; she reverted to her old behavior when she returned home. He decided to have her committed to a mental hospital.

Fortunately, before she was committed, her brother, who was a physician, began to suspect that her disorders were allergy-related. He took her to Dr. Randolph in Chicago for treatment. The first night in Chicago, the brother lit a gas range to prepare dinner, and immediately the woman began to exhibit symptoms. She complained of the gas, her cheeks got flushed, and she could hardly speak. She fell into a stupor and was unconscious for six hours. A neurologist who examined her said, "Impression: cataleptic attack. I would strongly suspect hysteria."

Dr. Randolph discovered, however, that the cause of her symptoms was that "she was exquisitely sensitive to utility gas exposure. In retrospect, many of her previous problems, from the time that she dropped plates as a child to her most recent attacks, could be traced to gas exposures."

Dr. Randolph also found that she was highly sensitive to other chemicals, especially pesticides, which accounted for her allergies to certain fruits. He found that it was not the fruits but the pesticides that evoked the allergic reactions and that she could eat these same fruits if they were organically grown.[4]

Oil heat may also create problems due to fumes from the furnace. If you use oil as a fuel source, it is best to have the oil burner separated as much as possible from your living quarters. In an apartment building, for example, choose an apartment on an upper floor.

The least offensive heating systems are electric or solar-powered units. Electric ovens and stoves are also preferable.

ELIMINATE HOUSEHOLD CHEMICALS

Dr. Marshall Mandell explains why environmental allergies are such a large problem in the United States:

Why should a person be allergic to anything that he eats, drinks, or inhales? After all, everything with which he comes into contact is derived in some form from something that is part of our Earth. The answers, we have discovered, involve mankind's increasing inability to cope with natural as well as unnatural substances in his environment.

How did this happen? For hundreds of thousands of years during the course of human evolution, changes occurred more slowly in man's natural environment than they do in the rapidly changing chemicalized and polluted world of today. ... Man had sufficient time to adjust to the pollution that resulted from a natural occurrence on his planet. ... He slowly evolved over a period of hundreds of thousands of years. He adapted. He survived. ...

During the past two centuries alone, man has brought such drastic change in his natural environment that it has become unnatural. When organic chemistry began in the nineteenth century, a whole series of combinations of chemicals were created that were never found naturally in the environment. Pesticides, herbicides (weed killers), insecticides, waxes, preservatives, colorings and additives, although they did the job they were designed for, contaminated the environment and filled man's body with residues that were totally alien to the human system. ... In short eveything man eats, drinks or inhales is now polluted with chemical agents that are foreign to his chemistry, and he is suffering the consequences of possessing a body that is incapable of handling the by-products of his amazing chemical technology.[8]

The result of our amazing chemical technology is the overloading of our immune systems, which are breaking down under the strain. The results are allergy and disease.

For this reason it is of primary importance to take whatever steps you can to eliminate as many chemical substances from your environment as possible.

Eliminate the use of household chemicals such as mothballs, detergents, furniture polish, toilet cleaners, air fresheners, scented soaps, shampoos, flavored toothpastes, and pesticides. At first this suggestion may seem to imply that one cannot clean one's home at all. However, there are a number of safe alternatives.

Lemon juice may be used for cleaning metals such as brass, aluminum, and copper. White vinegar will clean bathroom tiles. Baking soda can be used for a variety of cleaning purposes or as a room deodorant. It can also be used in place of toothpaste and as a mouthwash.

Several herbal toothpastes are available to replace the artificially flavored and colored ones ordinarily in use. A number of herbal shampoos can be purchased as well. You can make your own shampoo using two eggs plus two tablespoons of vodka.

The proper home furnishings may also be important to the allergic individual. In general, it is best to avoid synthetics (e.g., plastic, Naugahyde, and vinyl). Instead, use furniture made of organic materials, such as metal, wood, and canvas. Plastic lampshades should be removed, and venetian blinds should be replaced with shades made of natural fibers like cotton or wool.

Plastic turns up not only in furniture but also in other household items, as well in kitchen dishes and plastic wrap. It may be a good idea to replace plastic wrap with wax paper or to seal food in non-plastic storage containers. Use containers made of glass, china, and metal, not plastic.

AIR QUALITY

If you are suffering from environmental allergies and live in a highly polluted area, it may be advisable for you to move or take frequent trips to the country if possible. If you are "addicted" to city life, or if you simply don't want to or cannot move, you should use an acti-vated-carbon filter to at least keep the air within your home relatively allergen-free.

Smoking should not be permitted in your home. Recent advisory statements by the surgeon general warn that "passive" cigarette smoking can be as harmful as smoking itself. In addition to tobacco fumes, you may also be exposing yourself to the myriad chemicals the go into the manufacturing of cigarettes and the growing of the tobacco, such as the kerosene used to treat leaves, pesticides, and cadmium.

Like most people, you probably spend one-quarter to one-third of your time in the bedroom. So take special care to make this room as pollutant-free as possible.

Consider removing carpets and rugs. They can trap dust; the synthetic materials used in many carpets may aggravate the chemically sensitive. In general, get rid of synthetic materials here, as in other parts of the home. Be sure your blankets and sheets are made of cotton or flannel. You may also use wool blankets if you are not allergic to wool. It is best to use a cotton-filled or down pillow (unless you're allergic to feathers) and to avoid foam rubber.

Also avoid keeping throw pillows, stuffed animals, dolls, or any other small objects in the sleeping place; these tend to gather dust.

Dust and vacuum frequently. If feasible, have someone else do the vacuuming. If this is not possible, wear a filter mask when you clean your house.

As much as possible, keep books, magazines, and newspapers out of the bedroom; many individuals are sensitive to printed matter, particularly newsprint. Refrain from keeping perfumes, scented tissues, and cosmetics in the bedroom. In addition, since new appliances may emit odors for up to a year, they should also be stored outside the bedroom.

You might also want to put an air purifier in the room. It is important that the purifier be adequate for the size of the room. If it is not, the contaminants will not be stored properly but will be released.

The temperature of the bedroom should remain fairly constant through the night since for some individuals a change in temperature may trigger allergic reactions.

AVOIDING ALLERGENS

Reducing your exposure to chemicals in the workplace is more difficult than it is at home. In many offices and factories, exposure to chemicals and synthetic materials is inevitable. If changing jobs is impossible, attempt to reduce such exposure as much as possible. Not only industrial situations but modern offices also pose many problems for the allergic individual. There are fumes from copy machines, carbon paper, correction fluid, typewriter ribbons, and cleaning solutions. The cigarette smoke and perfumes of co-workers may also cause problems. Politely request that they refrain from smoking in your area, and bring in an air purifier. Request that chemicals not be used to clean your work area, or offer to assume responsibility for your own cleaning.

As far as office supplies go, whenever possible choose the lesser of two evils. Use standard carbon paper instead of carbonless paper, and correcting tape instead of correcting fluid. When using glue, a glue stick is preferable to rubber cement. It is also a good idea to avoid handling freshly made copies from the copy machine and not to accumulate empty bottles of copier fluid. Instead, the bottles should be placed in sealed trash containers and disposed of as quickly as possible. Avoid handling copier fluids. If you must handle them, do so only while wearing a mask and gloves.

OF COMPUTERS AND CARS

If you work with a video display terminal (VDT), that may also pose a problem. VDTs have been found to cause vision problems, headaches, dizziness, and fatigue. These reactions are thought to be due to the positive ions of the terminal screen, which draw negative ions from the nasal membranes – a change that affects the entire body.

If you use a VDT, it is advisable to keep a nearby window open or to circulate the air with a fan. Work, if possible, with a detached screen.

Cars are another source of environmental problems for many people with allergies. First, cars draw fumes from other vehicles on the road, so make sure yours has a valve to shut off outside air. It is best to have push-button windows so that all windows can be closed rapidly when entering a polluted area.

Avoid vinyl upholstery; use leather if it is available. If not, rayon is the second-best choice, and nylon the third. Remove rubber floor mats.

When buying a new car, test drive it and notice if you develop any allergic symptoms.

THE EFFORT IS WORTH IT

At first, all these changes in your environment may sound rather drastic. Indeed, they will take a lot of planning and time to carry out. But clinical ecologists believe that for some allergic individuals, the health benefits of such changes may make the effort well worth it.

CHAPTER FIVE

Allergy Tests

TESTING BY THE TRADITIONAL ALLERGIST

If you were to be tested for allergies by traditional means, your physician would use one of two types of tests: either the scratch test or the RAST.

In the *scratch test*, the physician puts a small amount of a stock allergen extract on a needle and then scratches the surface of the skin. If the skin becomes red and irritated, this means that you are allergic to that allergen. The problem with this test is that it detects only immune-mediated (IgE, IgG) allergies at best; at worst, it is not even very accurate at detecting these.[1]

The other traditional test, the *RAST* (the radio-allergo-sorbant test) is equally unreliable. In it your physician takes a blood sample and sends it to a lab, where it is tested to determine how IgE levels vary in response to different allergen extracts.

Neither of these tests can be used to detect nonimmune-mediated allergies, which have symptoms like hyperactivity, migraine, tension-fatigue syndrome, or mental illness.[2] Clinical ecologists believe that these allergies constitute 95 percent of all allergies.

TESTING BY THE CLINICAL ECOLOGIST

Clinical ecologists approach allergy testing in different ways from traditional allergists. The first difference is in the way the clinical ecologist looks at your case history. If you go to be tested, both the traditional allergist and the clinical ecologist will take your case history. This will involve the types of questions that you find on most medical questionnaires, plus some questions relating specifically to allergy, such as when your symptoms generally occur, if there is a history of allergy in your family, and if you have any other allergies. The clinical ecologist, however, is apt to put a greater emphasis on the case history and to be more rigorous in the questions he or she asks. This only stands to reason, since the ecologist takes a much broader view of allergy.

Accordingly, if you visit a clinical ecologist, you will be asked to give a detailed account of your diet. You will be asked how often you eat certain foods so that the clinical ecologist can find out if you are abusing them; you will be asked whether you crave certain foods, which may indicate an addictive-allergic reaction.[3] Many allergies are due to factors other than foods; so you may be asked whether you use gas or electric utilities and whether you feel better when you are in one place than in another. (Remember the case of the little boy who became vulgar at school but was fine at home.)

Since the clinical ecologist recognizes the role that allergy can play in almost any illness, he or she will be interested in your family's history not only of "allergy" but also of migraine, arthritis, or mental disease. If you bring in your child he may also want to know if any children in the family are hyperactive, have learning disabilities, or are bed-wetters.[4]

The clinical ecologist will also ask questions about your childhood, such as whether you were an overactive fetus (if you know) or if you caused your mother a difficult pregnancy. These episodes can sometimes correlate with the development of allergies later on in life. As a child did you have colic or rashes? Were you hyperactive, often ill, or a bed-wetter?[5]

The following symptoms in adult life may be equally indicative of allergies:

- digestive problems: diarrhea, constipation, bloating
- stuffy or runny nose
- stomachaches
- muscleaches
- fatigue

- mood swings
- depression
- compulsive eating, binges, or specific food cravings
- frequent or urgent need to void; difficulty urinating
- water retention with sudden weight gain of five to ten pounds.
- bed-wetting.
- dark circles, bags, or puffiness under the eyes
- flushed earlobes or cheeks
- coughing or wheezing
- intermittent loss of memory; difficulty concentrating
- headaches

THE INTRADERMAL PROVOCATIVE TEST

The intradermal skin test is a provocative test now widely used by both clinical ecologists and traditional allergists; it has replaced the scratch test for most physicians. Essentially it is an updated version of the scratch test; the allergy extract is injected rather than scratched into the outer layers of your skin. The test tends to be a bit more accurate at detecting immune-mediated allergies than is the scratch test or the RAST; but it is still not very reliable, nor does it objectively detect other types of allergies. When the test substance is injected into your arm, you should get a raised reddish-disk form at the site of the injection if you are allergic. This disk form is called a *wheal*. Its size is measured to determine your degree of sensitivity. For most traditional allergists, the testing stops there.

The clinical ecologist, however, is aware that most allergies do not manifest objectively (i.e., with a wheal or skin irritation) and therefore looks at subjective factors. For example, Dr. Doris Rap has her child patients make drawings both before the injection and after. Often these drawings are dramatically different. Videotapes prepared by Dr. Rapp show nice, well-behaved children transform when given the substance to which they are allergic. They start to whine, throw temper tantrums, crawl under furniture, cannot sit still, and are generally obnoxious.[7] For adults, handwriting samples may be taken.[6]

The clinical ecologist may also monitor your heart rate, temperature changes, and pupil dilation. You may be asked if your migraine or arthritislike symptoms recur. Your behavior is carefully observed.

The intradermal skin test is a form of provocative testing. It is the first step in determining the neutralizing dose, which turns off the symptoms as quickly as the provocative dose turns them on. On Dr. Rapp's videotapes the children revert back to normal when they are given the neutralizing dose.[8]

THE SUBLINGUAL PROVOCATIVE TEST

The sublingual provocative test is similar to the intradermal provocative test, except that instead of injecting the allergen extract, the physician places drops of one extract at a time under the patient's tongue – sublingually. It is not used by traditional allergists. Because sublingual absorption is very fast, symptoms may occur within a very few minutes after the extract is placed under the tongue. Sometimes the extract is administered without the patient knowing what the substance is, thereby eliminating the power of suggestion. It is often used to test for allergies to food dyes, which "tattoo" the skin if injected into an allergic patient.

Like the intradermal test, the sublingual test can be used both diagnostically and as a means of treatment. The patient's symptoms can be produced with one dilution of the allergen extract and eliminated with a different dilution of the same extract. Many patients find the sublingual test preferable to the intradermal test because it does not involve needles.

Both intradermal and sublingual provocative testing can be unpleasant at times, as well as initially expensive. These tests often precisely reproduce the symptoms of the allergy, so that if you get migraines, for example, you may get a migraine when you are given the substance to which you are allergic – not just a mild headache but a real migraine. It may also take a number of hours to determine the correct neutralizing dose for you, and this may be costly. But these are one-time expenses that may leave you symptom-free for the rest of your life without the use of harmful drugs or surgery.

APPLIED KINESIOLOGY

Applied kinesiology is a test widely used by alternative health care practitioners to determine the functioning of various body organs. It can also be used as a simple and inexpensive test for allergies.

Here's how it works. Your doctor asks you to fast on the day you are to be tested and to bring in samples of about twenty foods that you commonly eat. You may want to bring in some pure foods like milk, corn, or coffee to determine whether these foods are "no-no's" for you. Most of the foods – at least on the first testing – should, however, be in the form that you normally eat them. If you eat wheat as bread, bring in the bread you eat most frequently; if you never eat bread without butter, bring the butter. Sometimes you may find that you can eat foods individually but not together; it depends on you.

If you eat pizza often, bring in a small piece; or if you eat hero sandwiches, bring in a piece of one. Try to bring in samples that represent a fairly normal day's or week's consumption.

In applied kinesiology testing your physician will ask you to hold out your arm and then test it for its normal strength. You may be asked to extend it straight out or to the side. Then the doctor will push down on it and tell you to resist. That gauges your strength. The physician then begins to randomly test you by placing a small amount of the foods under your tongue and then asking you to resist as he tries to lower your arm. Usually you will be asked not to look at the foods being tested so that you do not consciously or unconsciously alter your response. The foods to which you are sensitive, even when merely placed under your tongue, will cause your muscles to weaken. Hence the doctor will be able to lower your arm much more easily.[9]

After this first test, you should alter your diet to eliminate the foods that made you weak. If they were combined foods like pizza, sandwiches, lasagna, or chow mein, simply eliminate those foods to start with and see how you feel for a week or two. If your symptoms do not clear up, you may want to test some foods in their pure form (e.g., wheat, dairy, or corn).

This test can be performed at home, so it can become something of a game, and an inexpensive game at that. You can test your family members, and they can test you for allergies to the foods you ate during the week. By playing around with this, you may discover what things are bad for you and create your own allergy-free diet.

CYTOTOXIC TESTING

Cytotoxic testing is by far the most controversial of the allergy-testing techniques. Most clinical ecologists do not even use it because it has been found to be unreliable. But those who attack clinical ecology often point to cytotoxic testing as proof that clinical ecology is nothing more than quackery. (This is discussed more fully in Chapter 6.)

In cytotoxic testing a sample of blood is drawn after you have fasted for twelve hours. The blood is sent to a laboratory, which puts drops of it on different slides. The blood is then exposed to different allergy extracts, and the reactions are viewed under a microscope to determine how many white blood cells have burst in response to a given extract. The lab technician then rates each response on a scale from 0 (no response) to 4 (a high degree of response).

One advantage of this test is that it is fairly inexpensive; over a hundred allergens can be tested with one sample of blood. It saves time for the patient, who merely has to supply the blood. However, the test receives very low marks for reliability from most physicians. Dr. Mandell, finds the test so inaccurate that he does not use it at all in his practice.[10] He has seen situations in which the same person's blood has been tested twice in less than a week and the results have been completely different. The test can as easily show false positives (saying that you are allergic to a substance when you are not) as false negatives (failing to detect an allergy). Part of this is because the test results depend in large part upon the interpretive skills of the lab technician and the fact that results may vary from technician to technician.

ALLERGY SMEARS   To perform an *allergy smear,* a technician examines a sample of the patient's blood, urine, stool, or bronchial secretions from the nose, eyes, or ears to check for eosinophils. *Eosinophils* are a type of white blood cell ordinarily found in the bloodstream. If there is a larger-than-normal percentage of them in one of the above substances, it may indicate an IgE-type allergy.

But this test is very general. For instance, it is useful in determining the presence of an allergy such as hay fever, but it does not help to identify the specific allergens. And it may not be positive in patients who have non-IgE-mediated allergies.

T AND B BLOOD CELL COUNT AND HELPER SUPPRESSOR RATIOS   This blood test checks the ratio to T to B cells, as well as the total number of T cells in the blood. If there are not enough T cells, or if the ratio of T to B cells is not in the normal range, it could suggest that the patient's immune system is not strong enough and may need strengthening. A weak immune system is often a contributing factor in the predisposition to allergy.

FASTING

Although total fasting can be performed on your own, it is highly advisable to fast under the supervision of a physician, who may wish to include this "test" with the others he performs. *Total fasting* means that the patient eats no food and drinks only glass-bottled water for several days. Typically, a fast to check for allergies will last four or five days. On the first day, and possibly on the second and third, the patient often does not feel very well because he is experiencing withdrawal symptoms from the foods he is not eating or drinking, especially the ones he has craved. By the fourth day the symptoms usually clear, and the patient generally feels better. At this point, the doctor may advise reintroducing one food per one meal at a time, instructing the patient to note whether certain ones cause symptoms.

Usually the patient first tests food that he neither loves nor dislikes. These are the foods to which he is probably not allergic. The foods should be eaten as the individual normally would eat them – cooked or raw. However, it is important to eat the foods in a plain state all by themselves, because a reaction to a seasoning, spice, dressing, or sauce on the food might be mistaken for an allergy to the food itself. The individual waits three hours; if no symptoms occur, he or she tests another food.

It is important to drink only spring water or distilled water while on a fast since many sensitive individuals are allergic to some of the chemicals in tap water. It is also a good idea to check the spring water itself (such as by applied kinesiology) to make sure it contains nothing to which the individual is sensitive. Again, the spring water should be in glass bottles since some people react to substances inside plastic bottles that are not inert and that can be released into water stored inside them.

Fasting is an inexpensive method of testing for allergies. It requires no special equipment and can be performed by the individual at home. Another potential advantage of fasting is that the fast itself may provide some rapid relief from allergic symptoms.

However, there are a number of drawbacks. First, many people find fasting very unpleasant. Second, fasting will not detect environmental allergies such as those to dust, mold, pets, and household chemicals.

Fasting is not for everyone. Those who are diabetic, hypoglycemic, malnourished, or chronically ill should not fast. Schizophrenics should only fast under medical supervision. If in doubt, check with your doctor.

THE COCA PULSE TEST

The *Coca Pulse test,* described in the case of Alex in Chapter 4, was developed in the 1930s by Arthur Coca, M.D., a pioneer in the field of immunology. He first discovered the efficacy of the test by working with his wife, who was suffering from severe heart pain. She had noticed that her pulse rate often sped up after eating. Dr. Coca suggested that she try taking one food at a time to see if particular foods were causing the effect. He found that certain foods, such as potatoes, provoked a rapid pulse, while others did not. When she avoided the foods that sped up her pulse, her heart pains disappeared. Coca began to use this test with his patients in 1956.[11]

You can perform the Coca Pulse Test at home. First, find your normal pulse range by taking your pulse every two hours. Then, on the test day, eat a different food every hour, beginning on an empty stomach in the morning. Check your pulse before eating and then again thirty minutes after eating. If it rises more than ten points, you may be allergic to the substance. Keep away from that specific substance for three days then test yourself again. Look for any symptom from increased pulse to lightheadedness.

A note of caution: Be sure you are not alone when such tests are done. The reaction could be sudden and severe.

KEEPING A FOOD DIARY

To perform the *food diary test*, write down everything you eat for one week, as well as the times at which you ate the foods. Concurrently, keep a record of your symptoms and when they occur. At the end of the week look back at the diary to see if any correlation can be made between eating a particular food and the onset of a particular symptom. For example, you might notice that you developed a headache every time you had wheat bread for breakfast. If you find a suspected allergen, eliminate that food from your diet and see if your complaint disappears. Then eat the food again to see if the symptom recurs. Suspected cause-and-effect relationships should always be confirmed.

The test requires no complex equipment, is inexpensive, and does not cause undue discomfort. However, it is a tedious job to record everything one has eaten, and some individuals may not keep accurate records. Also, if many foods are eaten at one meal, it may be hard to isolate which food is causing the problem unless each food in the meal is checked separately. In addition, you may not develop a reaction to the food immediately. Sometimes a reaction occurs a short while after eating the food, but at other times, especially if the reaction involves arthritis, bed-wetting, colitis, or ear fluid problems, the reaction is delayed for several hours. This makes it difficult to correlate the reaction with what has been eaten. If you are adept with a computer, however, you can easily find culprits using this method.

ELIMINATION DIETS

Dr. Rapp suggests two elimination diets. The first involves the elimination of one particular suspected food allergen until the symptoms clear. This may take anywhere from three to twelve days. After the elimination period, eat the test food all by itself on an empty stomach (that is, eat no food for four or more hours preceding the test). If you are sensitive to that food, symptoms usually occur within one hour of testing. However, sometimes the symptoms will not occur after the first time you eat the food; you may have to eat the food for two or three meals before you detect a reaction. And sometimes it is not only what you eat but how much you eat that causes adverse effects.

One problem with this method of testing is that if you are allergic to many foods, the procedure will take a long time to complete. However, the test is inexpensive, relatively easy to perform, and will pinpoint specific allergens.

Dr. Rapp's second elimination diet is the one-week elimination diet. Elminate for one week a number of the common foods to which many people are sensitive. For the entire week, avoid all dairy products, wheat, corn, eggs, citrus, sugar, chocolate, peanut butter, peas, food coloring, food additives, and preservatives. You should also eliminate all coffee, tea, cola, and tobacco. Dr. Rapp suggests that, if you experience an alleviation of symptoms after one week on the diet, you continue the diet for an additional week. At that point, if there is still no improvement, it is possible that your symptoms are not due to allergy, or that your food allergen has not been eliminated in the diet, or that your allergy is to environmental factors such as dust, mold, cooking gas, or household chemicals.

If there has been improvement by the end of the week (or two weeks), begin to add back the eliminated foods, one per day. For example, on Monday you might eat sugar cubes; watch to see if any symptoms develop. However, be careful not to add sugar-containing foods that contain other eliminated foods (e.g., wheat or eggs) as well. Chocolate milk would not be a good choice, for instance, because you might be reacting to the milk, the chocolate, or the sugar, and it would not be possible to tell which ingredient was causing the problem.

If symptoms do occur when you resume eating a test food, that food may well be an allergen and probably should be avoided in the future. It is advisable to recheck the food by eating it at five-day intervals to make sure that it was not a coincidence that symptoms developed the first time you resumed eating it. On subsequent days, try other foods that were eliminated, and watch for specific reactions to those foods. Different foods will cause different symptoms.

Dr. Rapp cautions that if you choose to follow the one-week elimination diet, you should not test foods that obviously cause severe allergic reactions. Also, adult individuals with serious reactions, such as asthma, and small children should test foods only under the guidance of a physician.[14] These individuals should not eliminate major foods or nutrients from their diets for more than one or two weeks without the supervision of a qualified physician.

Dr. Rapp notes that although an individual will often be able to correctly determine the major problematic foods by using the one-week elimination test, the allergy may be too complex to figure out without special help from a trained specialist. Individuals who have multiple food allergies plus a combination of inhalant and chemical allergies definitely need professional help, for hidden ingredients in the diet and unsuspected offenders in the home can be factors.

CHAPTER SIX

The Politics
of Allergy

To fully understand the political nature of medicine, I am going to give you a comprehensive picture of the methods and policies that are in the author's opinion used to suppress competing healing modalities.

If medical care in this country were provided in a free-market situation, this chapter would be unnecessary. However, due to the battle being waged against all forms of alternative health care by the American Medical Association (AMA) and other special interest groups and their supporters in the press and government, this chapter is necessary. Clinical ecologists are currently among the main targets of this battle. Many individual clinical ecologists are being harassed with the threat of losing their medical licenses.

I feel it is necessary also to be as comprehensive as possible, even at the risk of giving information that ostensibly seems irrelevant to the subject matter of this book.

However, if you feel that this lesson in medical history – which is really a lesson in the suppression of a therapy – is unnecessary, please feel free to skip over it. On the other hand, if you have been told that there is no relationship between your diet and how you feel, this chapter may prove valuable.

A LOOK AT MEDICAL HISTORY

In the early 1800s the practice of medicine in this country was in a sorry state. Bloodletting was the primary and preferred method of treatment by most physicians.

The belief prevailed among orthodox American physicians that a patient suffering from almost any disease could benefit from blood-letting. A prominent medical journal reported in 1837 that "among physicians there is no one remedy of greater importance in the treatment of disease than the lancet. In every part of our widespread country it is resorted to, and no adequate substitute can be found for its vast remedial powers."[1]

Indeed, Dr. Benjamin Rush, a leading nineteenth-century medical authority, advocated bleeding a patient for as long as the symptoms of the disease continued, until four-fifths of the patient's blood was drawn off and the pulse was weak and irregular. Rush, a professor of medicine at the University of Pennsylvania, advocated bloodletting as the remedy par excellence for those who were in a physically weak or even in a generally debilitated condition; it was used indiscriminantly on adults and children alike. If a patient was running a high fever and could not sit up without fainting, Rush taught that it was not safe – and therefore not good medical practice – to desist from bleeding the patient, even "if the pulse has ever so little tension on it."[2]

Bloodsucking leeches were almost as popular with American physicians as opening a vein. By 1856, one leech importer was bringing in 300,000 leeches annually; a competitor did an even brisker business, importing a half million leeches annually.

Another favorite remedy among American medical professionals was calomel, a laxative that is also known as mercurous chloride. It was used to treat all acute diseases, as well as syphilis and gonorrhea. Dr. Rush touted calomel as "a general stimulant and evacuant" and as "a safe and nearly ... universal medicine." He called it the "Samson" of medical substances. Physicians of that day prescribed calomel as a panacea for nearly all diseases, including epidemic cholera, venereal diseases, tetanus, yellow fever, smallpox, and rheumatism. Dr. Rush dosed his patients with enough calomel to produce four or five prodigious evacuations daily, then drew eight to ten ounces of blood with leeches to assure the optimal therapeutic effect.

Tooth decay and toothlessness were virtually universal in the 1800s. Coulter observes, "It is probably true that the toothlessness of many Americans was due to the doses of calomel they received from infancy, and this medication was doubtless responsible for many of the other ills described."[4] Endemic typhus, tuberculosis, malaria, and cholera, coupled with poor nutrition, poor personal hygiene, and the lack of adequate sanitation took a terrible toll on American health and lives.

The U.S. Department of War reported that the rejection rate of American volunteers for the Mexican War was twice as high as that of European and British recruits, owing to the failure of American volunteers to meet military standards for weight, robustness, and general health.

"The medical profession must take its share of the blame," writes Coulter, "for its failure to pursue an active search for safe and effective remedies and ... for its unbelievable maltreatment of patients with mercury, quinine, and bloodletting."[5]

It was against this backdrop that homeopathy began to gain acceptance in this country. Homeopathy is a system of medical practice developed by the German physician Samuel Hahnemann (1755–1843). He derived the word *homeopathy* from the Greek words *homion pathos*, meaning "similar illness."

Rebelling against the unscientific and often barbarous practices of orthodox medicine of his day – including bloodletting, leeching, and the gross, indiscriminate use of calomel – Hahnemann was attracted by Hippocrates's accounts of the cure or prevention of some diseases by the administration of substances known to produce effects similar to the symptoms of the disease. These remedial "similars" consisted of vegetable, mineral, or animal substances that, if given in large or repeated doses, produced in a healthy person symptoms similar to those manifested by sick patients.

Hahnemann decided to test the validity of treatment using similars by experimenting on himself. He took a strong dose of quinine, used to relieve the symptoms of malaria, and thereupon developed temporary symptoms of malaria. He concluded that the reason quinine relieved the symptoms of malaria was its ability to stimulate the body's natural immune response.

Emboldened by this discovery, he tested various medicinal substances on obliging friends and relatives. He kept a careful record of the symptoms the substances produced. These "provings" became the basis of Hahnemann's homeopathic method of treatment. His original sixty-eight provings grew to some six hundred by the end of the nineteenth century.

According to Coulter, who specializes in the history of homeopathy, Hahnemann formulated his findings into the "law of similars," which states that "each individual case of disease is most surely, radically, rapidly, and permanently annihilated and removed only by a medicine capable of producing [in the human system] in the most similar and complete manner the totality of [the disease] symptoms."[6]

Exasperated by the barbaric and ineffectual treatments offered by orthodox medicine, American physicians began to turn to homeopathy as a safe, gentle alternative. By the 1880's homeopathy had taken root and was successfully competing with orthodox medicine.

Homeopathy spread rapidly in this country and in Europe among the educated and the affluent; the establishmnt of homeopathic dispensaries was a boon to the poor, who were usually not charged. *The New York Times* commented that homeopathy "often cures when allopathy [traditional medicine] fails . . . . Whatever else it may be, it is not quackery. It has all the elements of a science."[7]

By 1900, almost 25 percent of all American physicians subscribed to the homeopathic discipline. It was taught in twenty-two domestic medical colleges. There were over a hundred homeopathic hospitals, and more than a thousand pharmacies across the country filled homeopathic prescriptions. Numerous homeopathic medical journals were published, and state homeopathic medical societies regulated the practice. In every respect, including licensing, the homeopathic physician enjoyed the same status as the traditional physician.

The rise of homeopathy shattered orthodox medicine's monopoly on health care. But the forces of orthodox medicine were not complacent. They were determined to eliminate homeopathic medical practice from the American scene.

In 1847 the American Medical Association was organized with the emplicit purpose of eliminating the practice of homeopathy in the United States.

The AMA called homeopathy a "delusion" and rigorously forbade physicians from consulting or consorting with homeopaths, regardless of the latter's medical expertise. In New York City the Academy of

Medicine excluded homeopaths from membership. The Connecticut Medical Society in 1852 summarily expelled some members of the Fairfield County Medical Society for practicing homeopathy. In 1873 the Massachusetts Medical Society, surrendering to AMA insistence, booted out eight homeopathic physicians who had held membership in the society for thirty years. The consequence of these expulsions – which *The New York Times* (June 7, 1883) called "unjust, unfair and abusive" – was that Boston became a hotbed of hostility toward the AMA.[8]

By 1865 the pharmaceutical industry fully supported the AMA's campaign against homeopathy. Since the homeopaths prescribed no proprietary medicines, they did not contribute to the manufacture and use of pharmaceuticals. Furthermore, homeopathic physicians actually discouraged the use of mass-produced, mass-marketed drugs in favor of an individual approach to illness.

By the turn of the century, the pharmaceutical industry's economic support of the AMA and its leaders was a fact. Prominent allopathic physicians were paid for endorsing specific proprietary medicines. By 1909 advertisements placed by pharmaceutical companies in the AMA's journal were the major source of the AMA's revenues. Coulter notes that out of 250 medical journals "published at the turn of the century ... only one was supported by the profession alone." The AMA journal itself reported that "practically all medical journals carry advertisements of proprietary remedies."[9]

The pharmaceutical companies deluged allopathic physicians with free samples of their products and sent out droves of public relations men who visited physicians' offices to praise their companies' products and to leave additional samples and gifts.

By such methods, the bond among the AMA, allopathic physicians and the pharmaceutical industry was cemented. The AMA, with its control over American medicine assured, used the revenues provided by its powerful ally, pharmaceutical industry, to prepare for the final assault on homeopathic medicine. Homeopathic medical schools were a primary target of the AMA when it formed its Council on Medical Education in 1904. The council's declared purpose was a noble one: to upgrade medical colleges. Unquestionably, medical colleges always need upgrading. But in retrospect, it is clear that the elimination of homeopathic medical schools was no small part of the AMA's purpose. One way to banish homeopathy was to get rid of the institutions in which it was taught.

The AMA planned to prove that homeopathic medical students were not as proficient as their traditional allopathic colleagues. However, this plan would have been impossible to implement. An AMA survey conducted in 1905 showed that 12 percent of allopathic graduates failed the medical-licensing examinations, compared with 3 percent of homeopathic graduates.

Raising admission standards and extending the medical school program to four years was not going to work, either. AMA studies of this showed that on the whole the caliber of students and teachers was higher at homeopathic schools than at conventional medical schools.

But the results of these studies spurred the AMA to devise a new rating system for schools. Its criteria would eliminate homeopathic schools from consideration for endowments and grants, on which medical schools depended (and still depend) for their existence. The rating system made a school's graduates' performance on state licensing examinations an insignificant criterion for the school's rating. Major significance was instead placed on the nature of the courses taught at the school, the elaborateness of its laboratories, and whether physicians teaching first- and second-year classes were employed full time at the school and whether they engaged in original research and published scientific papers in medical publications such as the AMA's journal. The most important criterion was whether the school was affiliated with a hospital and dispensary, the extensiveness of its libraries, and whether it maintained a museum of medical exhibits for students and faculty.

Both homeopathic and traditional medical schools protested the AMA's right to rate them, and they objected to the rigging of the criteria. In response, the AMA council brought in Abraham Flexner of the Carnegie Endowment, which was a primary source of funding for educational institutions.

The Flexner Report of 1910 embodied the AMA's unsolicited judgment of American medical schools. It was heavily influenced by the AMA's opposition to homeopathy. Flexner shared the AMA's bias; he saw no justification for the continued existence of homeopathic medical schools in the new age of "modern medicine."

Based on the Flexner Report and the AMA's school ratings, some state licensing boards barred homeopathic graduates from taking the licensing examinations. Andrew Carnegie, John D. Rockefeller, and other philanthropists accepted the AMA's recommendations and drastically cut their allocations to homeopathic medical schools. This occurred despite the fact that Rockefeller, who was ninety-eight when he died in 1937, never allowed any but homeopathic physicians to treat him.

Not long after, homeopathy began to feel the effects of the combined efforts of the medical establishment and the pharmaceutical companies to quash it. Without adequate funding, the number of homeopathic medical schools had dwindled to seven by 1918, and in 1928 the last one closed. This was the death knell for homeopathy.

TODAY'S MEDICINE

I have described in some detail the events leading up to the demise of homeopathy in order to illustrate how in my opinion the medical establishment deals with its adversaries. Homeopathy was not unique; it was merely the first in a long line of alternative methods of health care that the medical establishment singled out for elimination. The French saying *"Plus ça change, plus c'est la meme chose"* ("the more something changes, the more it remains the same") is particularly true of health care in America. Alternatives to traditional medicine constantly appear on the medical scene – for example, chiropractic, an alternative to traditional physiotherapy; chelation therapy, an alternative to heart bypass surgery; and anticandida and allergy-free diets and megavitamin therapy, alternatives to drugs and surgery for hyperactivity, arthritis, migraines, and mental disease.

One would think that the practice of medicine in this country would correspondingly change, that the medical establishment would look into these therapies, take what is valuable in them, and leave what is not. But this is not the case. Medicine, in terms of theory and doctrine, looks much the same as it always has.

However, medical care is becoming the largest industry in this country. As it stands now, we spend over $400 billion annually on medical care. This makes medicine the number-two industry in the country, second only to defense.

As the stakes grow, so do the number of players interested in maintaining the extremely lucrative status quo in the way the medical establishment treats and thinks about disease.

Basically, many of the characters are still around: the orthodox practitioners, the pharmaceutical companies, medical academia, and the AMA. Relatively new on the scene are special interest groups like the American Cancer Society and the Arthritis Foundation; government agencies like the Food and Drug Administration (FDA), the National Institutes of Health, and its parent agency, the Public Health Service; and various other industries like the food and chemical industries that also get involved when their interests are threatened.

Clinical ecologists now find themselves pitted against powers such as these. The pharmaceutical companies don't like them because they rarely use drugs, and because they speak out against prescribing them in other than emergency situations. In the author's opinion the orthodox medical establishment does not like clinical ecologists because they make the establishment look bad: clinical ecologists are able to cure many of the diseases that orthodox medicine deems incurable. Physicians find it easier and more time-saving to write out a prescription that will suppress symptoms than it is to spend an hour or two listening to patients' histories to determine what causes their illnesses.

The food industry's growth, like the drug industry's growth, has been built on certain accepted theories of health. So it is also a high-stakes player in the health care market. The food industry comprises such factions as the beef, dairy, and citrus lobbies, who understandably do not favor clinical ecologists' suggestions that many people are allergic to their products.

When studies are published that do not support their interests, fear for their profits causes these diverse and extensive monopolies to band together to defend their territory and preserve themselves from extinction.

That practitioners who advocate the "unconventional" theories of allergy are ostracized is hard to deny. Some doctors who receive their training from conservative institutions like the Harvard Medical School are becoming concerned about the negative impact of the marriage of politics and medicine on clinical ecology. One such doctor is Dr. Richard Podell, an allergist practicing in New Jersey.

"What should really be a scientific debate over how you treat food allergy and food sensitivity has become something of a political debate," he says, "something of a fight between several different doctor organizations, much like labor unions disputing their turf."[10]

A serious problem for clinical ecologists is that their articles are not being published in the top-notch medical journals. Although we may think that scientific research is objective, in reality the majority of articles published are those that support the status quo. Physicians are therefore not being exposed to many new ideas. The same material and authors are recycled over and over again. I believe one of the reasons that clinical ecologists may have trouble getting their articles published in these journals is that, as noted above, advertising by the drug companies often represents a substantial proportion of a journal's revenues. Hence, either expressly or tacitly, the pharmaceutical companies play a significant role in what gets published and what does not. As a result, many important studies are never seen or properly acknowledged, and vital work in the field of clinical ecology is being disregarded.

States Dr. Podell, "We have a number of occasions where articles have been written about nutrition or about allergy with a food allergy slant ... where it gets rejected with comments that are basically vicious.[11]

Thus on the one hand, studies showing the benefits of clinical ecology are being met with hostility, while on the other, the medical establishment maintains that there is no proof that clinical ecology has any merit. This sort of Catch-22 reasoning is not unique to the case of clinical ecology. Researchers who have found benefits in the use of vitamins, for example, experience the same thing. Although he has been awarded two Nobel Prizes for his work, Dr. Linus Pauling still has trouble getting his work published by the top journals. Dr. Pauling recounts one such experience with *The Journal of the American Medical Association* (JAMA):

On March 10, 1975, the AMA issued a statement to the press with the heading "Vitamin C will not prevent or cure the common cold." The basis for this quite negative statement was said to be two papers published on that day in the *Journal of the American Medical Association* (Karlowski, et al., 1975; Dykes and Meier, 1975). . . . The results observed by . . . some other investigators were not, however, presented. Despite their incomplete coverage of the evidence, Dykes and Meier concluded that the studies seemed to show that vitamin C decreases the amount of illness accompanying the common cold. . . . Thus their review of the evidence did not provide any basis for the AMA statement that vitamin C will not prevent or cure the common cold.

In order to present to the readers of the *Journal of the American Medical Association* (JAMA) an account of all the evidence, I at once prepared a thorough, but brief analysis of thirteen controlled trials and submitted it to the editor on March 19. He returned it to me twice with suggestions for minor revisions, which I made. Finally on September 24, six months after I had submitted the article to him, he wrote me that it was not wholly convincing and that he had decided to reject the article and not publish it in *JAMA*.

It is my opinion that it is quite improper for the editor of JAMA (or any other journal) to follow the policy of publishing only those papers that support only one side of a scientific or medical question and also to interfere with the proper discussion of the question by holding a paper that had been submitted to him for half a year, during which period, according to accepted custom, the paper could not be submitted to another journal.[12]

Dr. Pauling's latest fiasco involved his work on vitamin C and cancer. This time the publication was *The New England Journal of Medicine.* Dr. Pauling had been involved in two separate studies on the effects of vitamin C in reducing pain and prolonging life in cancer patients. The first study was performed in Scotland; the second, which essentially confirmed the first, was published in Japan. Both these studies showed, according to Dr. Pauling, that vitamin C did have beneficial effects in treating cancer patients.

The Mayo Clinic in this country then conducted its own studies, one in 1979 and the second in 1985. Based upon these studies, the National Cancer Institute and the reporter for the second study "announced vigorously that this study showed finally and definitely that vitamin C has no value against advanced cancer and recommended that no more studies of vitamin C be made."

What was not announced, according to Dr. Pauling, was that:

In our studies the vitamin C patients took large amounts of the vitamin without stopping, for the rest of their lives or until the present time, some for as much as fourteen years. In the second Mayo Clinic study ... the vitamin C patients received the vitamin for only a short time (median 2.5 months). None of the vitamin C patients died while taking the vitamin (somewhat less than 10 g per day). (The spokesmen) who commented on it both suppressed the fact that the vitamin C patients were not receiving vitamin C when they died and had not received any for a long time (median 10.5 months.[13]

Commenting on the politics behind these findings and the manner in which they were published, Dr. Pauling says:

When this Mayo Clinic paper appeared, January 17, 1985, Cameron and I were angry that Moertel and his Mayo Clinic associates, the spokesman for the National Cancer Institute and also the editor of The New England Journal of Medicine had managed to prevent us from obtaining any information about their results until a few hours before publication. Six weeks earlier Moertel refused to tell me anything about the work, except that their paper was going to be published. In a letter to me, he promised that he would arrange for me to have a copy . . . before publication . . . .

It is not often that unethical behavior of scientists is reported. . . . Improper representation of the results of clinical studies, as in the second Mayo Clinic report, is especially to be condemned because of its effect in increasing the amount of human suffering.[14]

In summary, most articles offering an alternative method of health care seem to suffer this fate when their authors try to get them published: The article is refused by the top-notch medical journals, often with a letter that is hostile or obtuse. When the alternative practitioner then seeks other channels to communicate the article's findings, he or she is labeled a quack or a charlatan, based on the fact that no articles in the top medical journals support their claims. Then, articles disproving the alternative claims are readily published, even though these articles are often based on studies that are fatally flawed. In the case of Dr. Pauling, for example, the article published claimed to duplicate Dr. Pauling's cited studies, when in fact much smaller doses of vitamin C were administered and the patients stayed on the vitamin for a shorter period than in Dr. Pauling's studies.

Dr. Doris Rapp agrees that politics creates barriers for new ideas. "They are not only not reading the literature; many of them won't look at the evidence," she says of the medical establishment. "There are many doctors across the United States saying the same thing, and

they're still saying that these are new ideas that aren't proven. . . .
Whenever someone comes up with something that's a little bit different
than what's in vogue right now, they're suspect."[15]

Dr. Rapp says that the published studies that claim to disprove the
work of clinical ecologists contain major and recurrent errors. For example, investigators often fail to choose patients who are sensitive to
the allergen being tested at the time when they are tested. Often, insufficient amounts of the allergen are fed to the patient. Placebos or
test foods may be coated in chocolate, or cookies containing wheat,
eggs, milk, and chocolate may be given to test for food colorings. If
the patient is allergic to any of these substances, a proper test is not
being made of his or her reaction to the test substances.

Confident that their treatments work, clinical ecologists often extend open invitations to members of the establishment to come and
see for themselves. Dr. Mandell, for example, who believes that 80
to 90 percent of arthritis cases are allergy-related, says that he has in-
vited the Arthritis Foundation to come and see his results but that it
consistently ignores the invitation. He says that he has asked them "to
send their highly qualified observers to an ecology unit with complete
freedom of access to the patients, the nurses, the charts and see for
themselves that arthritis is a reversible disorder. When we can show
that we can predictably stop the symptoms and predictably bring them
on and we can put the patient in a position of being able to be either
sick or well by having the knowledge that is available for many of them,
we're not talking about a mysterious illness for which there is no known
cause or no known treatment."[16]

The special interest groups involved in research into these diseases
are not content merely to ignore alternative therapies like clinical
ecology. Not only do they refuse to look into the merits of the therapies
in any responsible manner, groups like the American Cancer Society
and the Arthritis Foundation systematically attack them. One of the
techniques they use is to pinpoint a weakness in the therapy and then
emphasize that in an attempt to discredit the whole therapy. Neutraliz-
ing-dose therapy, for example, has no scientific explanation. It has been
shown to work, but no one knows how or why. The position of clinical
ecologists in this regard is that if a technique that is safe and nontoxic
has been shown to treat illnesses that may be either untreatable by

conventional means or treatable with toxic drugs, it is more important to safely heal the patient than to know how it works. The medical
establishment, on the other hand, will cite neutralization therapy as
unscientific and unproven, and from that premise it will label all of
clinical ecology unscientific and its practitioners quacks and charlatans.
The non sequitur in this reasoning should be apparent; just because
we do not know how something works does not mean that it does not
work.

Another object of attention of the critics of clinical ecology is
cytotoxic testing (see Chapter 5). This testing method is only about
50 percent accurate, and hence most clinical ecologists do not even
use it. Nevertheless, those opposed to clinical ecology cite cytotoxic
testing and conclude that the diagnostic techniques of clinical ecology
are inaccurate and unscientific. In fact, most clinical ecologists use
the same testing procedures and stock allergen extracts that traditional
allergists use; the differences are that clinical ecologists analyze test
results much more extensively by broader criteria, and they may use
sublingual rather than intradermal testing.

The public, little aware of the role that vested interests may play
in the health information they receive, is led to believe that the groups
speaking out against clinical ecology are objective and acting in the
best interests of health care. However, when vested interests speak out
vehemently against new treatments that are inherently harmless and
give unqualified approval to harmful, expensive, and possibly lethal
treatments (often involving drugs and surgery), their concern for the
public's well-being has to be questioned by this author.

Alternative health care practitioners who are fed up have finally
begun to come forth and ask the obvious question: Why is there such
resistance to employing nontoxic approaches when many harmful
therapies continue unchallenged?

MEDICINE AND MONEY

Dr. Richard Podell believes that alternative treatments are not dis-
missed simply because of disbelief or disinterest. "It's a matter of old-
fashioned economic competition," he says. "I don't think it's all

political. I think a lot of it has to do with the fact that most of these methods don't turn a profit for anybody."[19] Many alternative methods of therapy are based on dietary manipulation or vitamins, which are naturally occurring substances and therefore unpatentable. Accordingly, the profitability of the "patent" drugs is lacking in these therapies.

Dr. Ralph Moss, co-author with Dr. Theron Randolph of *An Alternative Approach to Allergies,* explains that "drugs formed the basis for a large industry, which grew from small beginnings in 1950 to a huge business. American doctors wrote 120 million tranquilizer prescriptions a year in the late 1970s, enough for 12 billion doses. Prescription tranquilizers alone earned the drug companies $650 million a year. It is hardly surprising then that organized medicine took the path of drugging the patient, as opposed to the more difficult but more logical path of deducing the actual environmental causes of a patient's illness and then treating the problem by eliminating the causes."[20]

THE INFLUENCE OF THE FOOD INDUSTRY

For years now the food industry and the medical establishment have lived in peaceful coexistence. The food industry has been able to sell its products to Americans in just about any form without any serious challenges by the medical establishment as to the health consequences or nutritional value of the foodstuffs. When unruly groups like clinical ecologists appear on the scene to upset this balance, food and medicine band together in a mutually advantageous alliance. The food industries may, for example, give generous research grants to individuals, institutions, and groups interested in disproving that food additives cause hyperactivity in children. Food additives make otherwise unpalatable-looking food appear appetizing, they prolong shelf life often indefinitely, and they make mass-marketing possible. All these factors operate to increase profits and facilitate marketing. Food additives are just one example, of course. Unless the evidence is absolutely overwhelming and the public has already made a shift in belief on its own, the food industries have no trouble finding spokespeople for its products. As Dr. Rapp points out, even now, ten years after Dr. Benjamin Feingold made the public aware of the connection between food coloring and hyperactivity in children, the latest pediatric journals are still insisting that food colorings cause hyperactivity in children only rarely.

Dr. Moss says: "Orthodox allergists focused their attention on pollens, dusts, molds, and danders, which can produce dramatic and measurable reactions in sensitive individuals. But, pollen and dusts are politically innocuous; one can criticize them as much as one likes, with few repercussions. Foods, however, especially the common ones, form the basis of powerful, interlocking financial interests. To name corn, wheat, milk, eggs and beet and cane sugars as the sources of illness, even in a minority of the population, will not make friends among the commercial producers of these foods."[21]

The food industry has good reason to be concerned. Environmental medical experts agree that many people have intense allergies to beef, citrus fruits, and milk. Meanwhile the meat, dairy and cirtrus industries spend enormous amounts of money to convince the public and the American Dietetic Association that their products are an essential part of every diet. They claim that beef is the best source of protein, that milk is needed for calcium for strong teeth and bones, and that orange juice provides our vitamin C requirements. These claims however, are far from true.

When we rely on beef for protein, we also take in large amounts of saturated fats, uric acid, and residues from the drugs used to keep these animals from infection and disease in their unsanitary surroundings. Some physicians warn that antibiotic levels in beef and chicken are so high that they can render ordinary antibiotics ineffectual when we are really sick and need them to fight off infection. Only now, with the myriad diet and health books warning of the hazards of eating too much red meat, is the medical establishment parroting these warnings.

Another food industry fallacy promoted by the medical establishment is that we need milk to supply adequate calcium. Many people are allergic to milk, and this allergy can interfere with proper calcium absorption. Green leafy vegetables and sesame seeds, for example, are high in calcium and are easily digested so the calcium is properly absorbed.

Orange juice is rich in vitamin C, but because of the massive advertising around it, many people have "abused" it and are now allergic. All fruits and vegetables supply vitamin C in varying amounts, and a diet rich in a number of them will provide as much vitamin C as orange juice. I always take a vitamin C supplement even when I eat lots of fruits and vegetables because of its important role in detoxification and strengthening the immune system.

Lendon Smith, M.D., a renowned pediatrician and nutritional physician, says he is embarrassed about the prevailing ignorance among doctors of the role that food plays in health. To demonstrate that old myths die hard, he points out that his son, who attended medical school twenty years after he did, was given the same conservative and brief information on nutrition. According to Dr. Smith, doctors are trained to be good diagnosticians, but it stops there.[22]

OVERLOOKING THE OBVIOUS

Yet even these "good diagnosticians" are baffled by such nervous system reactions as the tension-fatigue syndrome, despite numerous books and articles written by reputable clinical ecologists.

For example, on three different occasions during the early 1970s, review articles appeared in a leading pediatric journal, *Pediatrics*, describing groups of pale children with circles under their eyes who complained about abdominal pain, headaches, and muscle pains. In each article the symptoms were attributed to emotional or psychogenic causes. The diagnosis of food allergy was never seriously considered, and no attempt was made to place these children on diagnostic elimination diets.

In response to one of these articles a group of clinical ecologists wrote, "The authors' resistance to treat by dietary manipulations ... is a terrible oversight at the very least. Because allergy patients do have these symptoms (abdominal pain, leg ache, pallor, etc.) we cannot disregard them and hope they will go away, as is implied by the authors. What is not looked for certainly in many instances, will not be found. ... "During the past several years, we've seen 94 children with the tension-fatigue syndrome caused by food allergy. ... We suggest that patients with similar symptoms be given the benefit of an elimination diet before attributing their symptoms to functional or emo-tional causes."[23]

It is mind-boggling that the majority of pediatricians would not consider a child's diet, not to mention an adult's, as a probable cause of lack of well-being.

According to Dr. Mandell, highly qualified physicians such as Drs. Randolph, Rinkel, Philpott, and Coca have begun to openly question the routine practices of such physicians – and not in pediatrics alone. Says Dr. Mandell, "There is a great (and often heated) debate going on among the members of the medical community, a kind of old ver-sus new school debate. The physicians who continue to practice the conventional symptom-relieving, drug-oriented medicine they were taught in medical school (and which is still being taught in medical schools by the same team of old-guard defenders) are in conflict with the doctors who are more oriented toward discovering the cause of a problem, doing something about it, and eliminating the need for medication."[24]

No one gets well by diagnosis alone. Proper treatment is essential. The clinical ecological approach to treatment employs what appears to be common sense: The least invasive therapy should be utilized be-fore the more radical, potentially harmful ones, and treating the cause of a disease is preferable to masking its symptoms.

But the obvious is not so obvious if you have been conditioned to see differently.

A FULL-SCALE WAR

Unfortunately, what is ultimately a mother of scientific inquiry has escalated into a full-scale war of egos and economics. Clinical ecologists have published numerous articles in their own Journal supporting the continued use of sublingual and subcutaneous neutrali-zation techniques in the treatment of food allergies. Yet a report issued in July 1984 by the American Academy of Allergy and Immunology Committee on Adverse Reactions to Foods held that "after careful consideration of the available data, the American Academy of Allergy issued a series of position statements in which the opinion was expressed that sublingual (under the tongue) and subcutaneous neutralization techniques should be considered unproved and should be reserved for experimental use only in well-designed trials."[25]

In the opinion of Dr. Podell, the reports sponsored by this premier academic allergy organization were based on inadequate evidence. But as a result of this statement, the Department of Health and Human Services has decided that these therapies are no longer acceptable for insurance coverage. This was further assisted by active lobbying of the federal government and insurance companies and of the participating physician organizations, and by the efforts of the American Academy of Allergy and Immunology to discredit claims of effectiveness by clinical ecologists. According to Dr. Podell, this measure was announced during the month of August, when most physicians and patients were vacationing. Physicians and patients had only thirty days to protest. The academy had hoped that their action would receive little response or resistance. Even though more than ten thousand letters protesting this proposal were received, most health insurance companies no longer cover neutralization therapy. Unfortunately, insurance coverage has a huge impact on the type of treatment the public chooses. Although patients may wish to receive neutralization therapy because it has been shown to work in similar cases, they may be forced either to discontinue treatments or to choose a more expensive, more toxic, and less effective treatment but one that is covered under their health insurance policies.[26]

The conscious efforts of orthodox medicine to control and maintain a monopoly on approved medical practice has succeeded to date by this multifaceted approach.

RESISTANCE TO CHANGE

The course of medicine today is guided by the peer-review system, in which doctors basically stand in judgment of their colleagues. This may seem as it should be, that only doctors are in the position to adequately evaluate the claims of other doctors. But it is not necessarily true. For example, biochemists are qualified to structure and interpret tests on the effects of foods and vitamins. Scientists in general are in a position to verify whether a study as performed adheres to proper procedure and follows its own protocol.

The peer-review system creates many conflicts of interest. Often, a "buddy system" exists, in which doctors who edit the major medical journals or who head the top medical universities and organizations continually favor the work of colleagues who hold the same beliefs that they do. This buddy system also extends outside the medical establishment itself, where doctors who hold the "right" beliefs move to high-paying positions, like chairmen of the boards of the industries they have supported while holding government agency positions. These lucrative incentives, together with the tendency of researchers to favor work that reflects their own ideas, often shuts out innovative ideas and techniques, as well as ideas that come from outside the academic mainstream, such as, of course, the contributions of clinical ecologists.

"Personally" says Dr. Podell, "I think that if one were to lay down all the studies end to end and consider them outside of the political context, outside of whose economic well-being is at stake, I think one could quickly get to some reasonable conclusion. Where there is uncertainty, one could do the studies rather quickly to resolve these uncertainties. The important point is that's not being done. It's being waged as a political battle instead."[27]

Money, politics, and ego are not the only factors that conspire to paralyze medical knowledge. Tradition and insecurity also come into play. As Dr. Mandell explains, "Respected teachers transmit a complex body of information and guiding principles to the medical students and neophyte physicians with whom they come in contact. Well-founded or not, right or wrong, deeply ingrained beliefs that were gained during a difficult and prolonged apprenticeship are not easily given up by those who have labored to acquire them; medical traditions are highly resistant to change once they have been accepted as facts."[28]

Dr. Philpott has a subtly different theory for their reluctance. "There's a lot of anxiety, not just in the people who have the disease, but in the doctors who handle them." In an attempt to resolve these anxieties, doctors set up schools of thought to protect themselves. According to Dr. Philpott, this is particularly seen in psychiatry. "There is almost a religious zeal for these schools of thought. So the doctor has his security, and he defends that. When he hears anything else, he either treats it with indifference or he attacks it. When it comes to change, you have to consider the personality of the people involved."[29]

Throughout medical history numerous therapies have been utilized long before anyone knew why they worked. For example, in 1740 the British Navy realized that including limes in the diets of men at sea prevented the onset of scurvy, a disease often fatal for sailors. This practice helped to save many lives before scientist Albert Szent-Gyorgi isolated vitamin C (ascorbic acid) as the antiscurvy ingredient. Such open-mindedness to new discoveries and treatments, however, predates our age of scientific bureaucracy.

The same is true of pellegra, which is referred to as the Disease of the Four D's: dermatitis, diarrhea, dementia (psychotic behavior), and death. Fortunately for those suffering from this dreadful disease, it was discovered, long before our medical bureaucracy set in, that it could be cured by niacin (vitamin B_3). There is little doubt in my mind that if this cure were found today, it would be rejected by the medical establishment as unproven, while at the same time it would spend millions of dollars to find a "scientific" cure. Indeed, Dr. Philpott and other nutritionally oriented psychiatrists have noted that the symptoms exhibited by mental patients suffering from pellegra encompass the range of known psychiatric disorders. Yet the medical establishment consistently rejects studies, even double-blind studies (such as those done by Abram Hoffer, M.D., and Humphrey Osmond, M.D.) showing the benefits of treating schizophrenic patients with niacin.

SCIENTIFIC BUREAUCRATS

In the medical industry there seems to be no shortage of scientific bureaucrats. Hundreds of people are on salary in leading universities and the government who have the training to execute proper studies, but in many cases their minds are closed. It would be ideal, of course, for these established powers to undertake joint studies with clinical ecologists. Unfortunately, there's a Catch-22 here: To get the bureaucrats' cooperation and research findings, clinical ecologists need a body of large-scale scientific results; to obtain those results, they need the cooperation and funding.

But such studies are essential. Even traditional allergists acknowledge that the biochemical mechanisms at work in the allergic-response syndrome are not fully understood. They are highly complex, and extensive investigation must be made of their root cause and reversal.

However, as Dr. Rapp states, "It seems that there's a reluctance on the part of the people who have the grants to do the research in this area. Clinicians such as myself are really not qualified to do the research. And even though I have videotapes, movies, and samples of the relevant results, this doesn't seem to make any impression on the powers that be in the field of medicine. The result is that the average doctor in practice doesn't even know that these newer methods of solving these problems exist."[29]

If, as it is estimated, one out of every eight to ten persons suffers from a major allergy, while roughly half of the general public has a milder allergy to certain foods, chemicals, or inhalants, then education of those "average doctors" clearly should be an objective of American medicine.

According to Dr. William Crook, "Even if we had ten times as many allergy specialists in America, we still wouldn't have enough to look after all the allergic patients." Yet, as he points out, the sad fact remains that "relatively little time and attention is devoted to allergy in medical school or in internship and residency training programs."[31]

As the Allergy Foundation of America has publicly stated, "There's no question that allergy has been sort of a stepchild of medicine, either ridiculed or ignored."[32]

EDUCATING THE PUBLIC

Since the medical schools are resistant to teaching new theories to young doctors, educating the public should be the immediate goal. As Dr. Rapp points out, "If we can get the people watching and emphasizing what caused the problem instead of running for the pill bottle, we'll make people better in the long run. They'll be less sick, and they won't need to go to the doctor as often."[33]

Doctors who care about long-term health are exactly what we need, and not just for altruistic reasons. Dr. Philpott warns, "The simple truth is that our country needs physicians who are interested in curing and preventing the cause of disease rather than merely in symptomatic treatment and relief. If we fail at this task, then the medical field will not be the third largest industry in our country as it is today, but the largest. If this tragedy occurs, and statistical analysis suggests it well might be by the year 2000, then it will take the entire Gross National Product to support its existence.[34]

With the medical schools resistant to teaching new theories to young doctors, the ball is in the public's court to start educating itself. Many of the books that are out on the market today on all sorts of different health and nutrition topics have been written by doctors who are fed up and frustrated with trying to get the medical establishment to take note of their findings. At least by writing these books they give the public the chance to judge for themselves whether a given therapy is worth their while.

It is also important that the members of the public begin to realize that they can learn to take care of themselves in many areas of health. Some people do not want the responsibility for taking care of themselves; they would rather have bypass surgery than cut down on meat and dairy and sugar products; or they would rather drink that extra coffee and smoke that cigarette, and let someone try to patch them up later. For these people the symptom-suppressing approach of modern medicine is adequate and in fact is just what they want. But not everyone is like that. There are people who would change in order to improve their quality of life if they had access to the information telling them how to do so. These are the real losers in the medical establishment's war on alternative health care.

The high cost of health care, coupled with the ever-increasing incidence of drastic illness (AIDS, cancer, osteoporosis), has raised insurance premiums across the board. It is not just the sick who pay. Family and friends see their loved ones wasting away; employers suffer the costs of high absenteeism. Each individual in society suffers from the ever-present fear that some dread disease will strike him or her next. Looking at this situation realistically, it is obvious that something has got to change. More megadollars spent in the way they are currently being spent are not the answer to anything, except to move medicine to the position of the largest industry in the nation.

Clinical ecologists certainly don't have all the answers; a tremendous amount of research remains to be done. But the validity of their findings so far is undeniable and hard to ignore. It is encouraging, therefore, to remember that historically, when orthodox medical practitioners could no longer ignore or deny the facts about a disease or therapy, they reevaluated their position and claimed the once-controversial research findings as their "new medical discovery."

It is a safe prediction, then, that the American Academy of Allergy and Immunology will shortly be reporting that non-IgE-mediated food sensitivities do exist. After that point, it is a matter of time once again before they accept the therapies that clinical ecologists have been using for years in the treatment of these (presently "nonexistent") sensitivities.

CHAPTER SEVEN

The Allergy-Free Diet

OVERVIEW

Like all aspects of allergy, the allergy-free diet that will bring you optimal health is an individual matter. No two people will have exactly the same reaction to the same foods or combinations of food. Whether you are now eating a healthy diet or are simply eating whatever comes along will determine whether adopting an allergy-free diet will mean minor adjustments or dramatic changes in your food regimen. Your current state of health will also be a factor. If you are healthy and normally full of energy but simply suffer from occasional fatigue, which you and your doctor have determined occurs after you have eaten a specific food, then you may simply eliminate that food, and that will be your allergy-free diet. On the other hand, if you suffer from chronic tension-fatigue syndrome resulting from multiple allergies to the staples in your current diet – say milk, wheat, and beef – your allergy-free diet will be substantially different from what your diet is now.

DESIGNING YOUR ALLERGY-FREE DIET

The optimal diet is one in which the foods come primarily from fruits, vegetables, and complex carbohydrates. Complex carbohydrates should be divided about equally between grains and legumes.

Many people are allergic to corn or wheat, so their diet will exclude them. But there are still many grains to select from – namely oats, barley, rye, millet, rice, tritical, amaranth, and buckwheat.

Legumes are not commonly responsible for allergies, except for soy, which is frequently used in many foods in the form of soy oil, soy sauce, or soy flour. They are much more varied than the grains, numbering in the fifties. Legumes that are readily available at most grocery stores or health-food stores include navy beans, black beans, lentils, split peas, chick peas (or garbanzo beans), lima beans, and black-eyed peas.

Also, your diet should include a few starchy vegetables like carrots, yams, squash, sweet potato, white potato (provided you are not allergic to it), turnip, parsnip, or burdock. In addition, you should try to eat three or four nonstarchy vegetables per day and one serving of sea vegetables like nori, wakambi, cambi, and arami. These vegetables are available at stores selling Oriental products and in most health-food stores. They are good sources of iodine, calcium, and protein.

Optimally, you should have two to four fruit servings a day, preferably not citrus (orange, grapefruit, lemon, or lime). It is not that these are not good for you; rather, they have been abused by most Americans as a result of massive advertising, and many people are allergic to them. All fruits must be thoroughly washed. Grapes, for example, in addition to being exposed to chemical pesticides, develop a yeast on the skin that can stimulate yeast infection in the intestine. Organic, locally grown produce is always the best. Many pesticides permeate the skin of the fruit or vegetable, and washing will not get rid of it; apples are a primary culprit here. Out of season, produce is brought into the country generally from Chile or Mexico, countries which do not regulate the use of pesticides, as does United States. Pesticides like DDT, which have been banned here, are commonly used on their products in large doses. Then we import the product and eat it.

It is especially important, if you are going on a limited diet or a fresh-food fast to cleanse the body, that you try your best to get organically grown produce, as you will at that time be particularly susceptible to toxins.

You should be drinking at least eight to ten glasses of water per day, depending upon the amount of exercise you do and the climate. Dehydration can lead to kidney problems, shrinkage of the brain, and constipation.

Your salt intake should be kept at a minimum, even if you do not exhibit a specific allergy to it. At first you may find that your foods just do not have any flavor, but after a week or so you will begin to develop heightened sensitivity to their natural flavors. Combining different foods (grains, legumes, and vegetables) and adding spices and garlic will enhance flavors. The cleansing and immune-stimulating powers of garlic are destroyed when you heat it, so I recommend that you press it freshly on to your foods after they are cooked. There are also a number of delicious salt-free or low-sodium spices available at many health-food stores. One of the tastiest lines is put out by Nile Spices.

Also important are the various types of sprouts, which are rich in enzymes—which aid digestion—as well as vitamins and minerals. The amount of vitamin C increases by as much as two to three hundred times between the seed and the full sprout. All sorts of sprouts are available commercially today: of course the alfalfa sprout—a favorite; the radish sprout, which is a spicy and delicious addition to a salad; the mung bean (or soy) sprout, which is used widely in Chinese cooking. Many health-food stores now carry lentil, pea, azuki bean, and other types of sprouts. They are all good, and you can use them in salads, sandwiches, vegetarian tacos, and other vegetable dishes. Essene bread is an unleavened bread made entirely of sprouted grains (no flour). It is packed with nutrition and provides a good alternative for those with allergies to ordinary bread (be it from the yeast or the flour). If you are allergic to wheat, make sure you buy a wheat-free variety of bread.

If you are allergic to wheat, corn, dairy, or sugar, I recommend that you find a good health-food store in your area and begin to experiment with the various products made without those foods. As the awareness of the prevalence of allergies to these foods has grown, so has the variety of sugar- , wheat- , dairy- , and corn-free products. There are, for example, delicious rice and barley flour or almond butter cookies sweetened only with fruit juices, which not only satisfy an urge for sweets but are also healthful and low in calories. These can be a good snack for children allergic to the ingredients in commercial sweets. Other foods you may want to try are rice cakes, a low-calorie substitute for crackers or bread; rye or rice breads, which are made without wheat (Food for Life puts out an especially good line); wheat-free granola cereals, good substitutes for regular cereals. If you are allergic to milk, you may want to try using the new coconut or almond milk juices on your cereal. These juices are readily available at most health-food stores and at many grocery stores.

If you are concerned about getting enough fiber but are sensitive to wheat, avoid wheat bran. This diet, high in fruits, vegetables, and complex carbohydrates, will give you all the fiber you need. Not only does this diet give you five to ten grams of fiber with each meal; in the case of barley, for example, you are also getting a blood-cholesterol-lowering agent. This is also true of garlic.

Ideally you should eat raw, uncooked foods as often as possible. Valuable enzymes that aid our digestion and assist in the scavenging of free radicals are destroyed by heat. This means eating lots of big salads with a variety of raw vegetables like red- and green-leaf lettuce, watercress, arugula, radishes, scallions, peppers (unless you are allergic to nightshades), and lots of sprouts. The spicy raw vegetables like watercress, arugula, and radish also work as anticandida nutrients and blood purifiers, much like garlic.

Some vegetables, however, are actually better utilized when cooked. Cooking breaks down the cells and makes the vitamins more easily absorbed by our bodies. Carrots, for example, are an excellent source of vitamin A (beta carotene), but they are more easily digested and absorbed when cooked. When you do cook your vegetables, do so only for a few minutes; they should be crunchy even when cooked, never soggy, and never overcooked. You can steam or lightly sauté them in a little vegetable oil (no corn oil if you are allergic to corn). Toasted sesame and peanut oil, available at health-food stores and Oriental markets, add a delicious nutlike flavor to vegetables. You can use a bit on steamed vegetables instead of butter or to sauté them. Vegetables that should be cooked for maximum vitamin absorption include cauliflower, brussels sprouts, asparagus, and broccoli.

ADEQUATE PROTEIN IN THE ALLERGY-FREE DIET

If you are allergic to milk, beef, or another food that now provides large amounts of protein in your diet, you are probably concerned that if you eliminate this food, you will become protein deficient. Much emphasis is placed on protein in the United States. Almost every time I tell someone that I am a vegetarian and eat no dairy products, the first question I am asked is, "How do you get your protein?"

A properly designed diet rich in complex carbohydrates and legumes, fruits and vegetables, will give you all the protein that you need to maintain optimal health.[1]

Contrary to what most of us have been led to believe, too much protein is actually harmful to your health.[2] For quite some time now, the myth has been that any excess protein that we eat is stored in the body for future use. Although this is true to the extent that excess protein may cause a faster turnover rate of proteins in the body, this is by no means beneficial. This faster metabolism of protein can cause certain cells to age prematurely, leading to acceleration of the aging process in the body in general.[3] Excessive protein intake also causes the body to produce urea, a waste product of protein metabolism. Large amounts of urea make the liver and kidneys overwork and can lead to damage of these organs.[4]

The other major myth we have received about protein is that animal products are our only reliable source of it, that they are the only "complete" source of protein. As much as the dairy and beef industries would like us to believe this, it is also not true. In fact, not only do animal products fail to have a monopoly on the protein market, they are not even our best sources of it.[5]

A LESSON ON PROTEIN The protein we eat contains twenty-three different amino acids; all are vital to our body. But of these, we need only worry about nine, because the body can manufacture the other fourteen by itself, provided our diet is healthy. The importance of consuming protein on a daily basis lies in its ability to supply us with these amino acids, which in turn are used for growth, maintenance, and repair of all parts of the body. Such life-sustaining substances as enzymes, regulatory hormones, antibodies, and hemoglobin (responsible for the transport of oxygen) are made up of protein. Collagen, the "glue" that holds individual cells together, is a protein. Without protein, we would literally fall apart.

Obviously, then, getting enough protein in our diet is important. Fortunately for those who are either allergic to animal proteins like milk and beef or who simply want to improve their health and well-being, protein comes in many forms.

THE NEWS ON PROTEIN   For over forty years now the buzzword when talking about protein has been *complete*. Complete proteins are those foods containing all the nine essential amino acids. Foods containing only some of the amino acids were called incomplete and thus incapable of meeting our protein needs. In the 1970s Frances Moore Lappé, in her book *Diet for a Small Planet*,[6] was among the first to present the public with a viable alternative to animal product proteins. Lappé showed that by combining certain foods, like rice and beans, chick peas and sesame seeds, peanuts and wheat, foods that were not in themselves "complete" proteins, they became so when properly combined. While this may have been a new concept to the American public, it in fact merely reiterated principles that had sustained life for thousands of years before we were talked into believing that we would become malnourished if we did not consume animal products. Many of the grain-legume combinations of the Middle East, Mexico, Central and South America, and India have been providing the protein requirements of people in these countries since the dawn of history.

So much for the myth that animal protein is the only source of protein. How about the myth that animal protein is our best source of protein?

THE NEW FOCUS ON QUALITY   Modern nutritionists are now playing down the theory of "complete" and "incomplete" protein and emphasizing the quality of a protein.

Quality is determined by how well a given food is utilized by the body for its requirements. The digestibility of a food, then, is an important factor because if we cannot digest it, we cannot use it, no matter how potentially rich it may be in protein.

To determine the quality of a food, the concept of *net protein utilization* (NPU) was developed.[7] This is a measure of how much protein we actually use from a given food.

Under the new criteria, researchers are discovering that many whole grains, seeds, fruits, and vegetables appear in a much more favorable light than do chemical-laden meats, for instance.[8]

As a protein source, eggs have the highest NPU; they are 95 percent utilized by the human body. Beef, however, is only about 70 percent utilized, which is only slightly above dried beans; these beans, combined with the right grain, will give you an even greater amount of utilizable protein than beef.

Ideally, then, eggs provide our most perfect form of protein. But there are many practical reasons why you may not or cannot use eggs as your sole source of protein. First, you may be allergic to them. If you are not now, you undoubtedly would develop an allergy later on if you ate eggs daily. Second, eggs are very high in cholesterol, which many people are trying to limit these days as a preventive measure against heart disease. Third, it would not be long before you just plain got sick of eggs. And fourth, your diet would probably become deficient in a number of nutrients that you would get by eating a varied diet.

The best way to get protein is from a wide variety of sources. That way you ensure an adequate intake not only of protein but also of a broad range of other nutrients required to maintain good health. This is one reason why food combining is so important. It provides you with the protein you need, and at the same time it gives you fiber from the carbohydrates and legumes—which is absent from animal proteins—together with a wealth of vitamins.

HOW MUCH PROTEIN DO YOU NEED?   Despite the protein hype that we have been getting for so long, most Americans actually consume much more protein than they need. Government statistics are as inflated for protein as their Recommended Daily Allowances (RDAs) are deficient for vitamins. The National Academy of Sciences actually adds a 30 percent "fudge factor" onto its protein estimates, which are inflated to begin with. These "beefed-up" figures say that men should get around 56 grams of protein daily and women 46 (calculated on the basis of .8 grams per kilogram of body weight.[9] A kilogram is equal to 2.2 pounds).

A more realistic calculation is based on the amount of nitrogen lost in protein metabolism. When we eat protein, some of it is replaced, some of it is broken down and resynthesized, and some of it is lost. Protein is our only available source of nitrogen. Thus when we lose nitrogen, we lose protein, and vice versa. By measuring nitrogen loss, the realistic protein requirement of a normal man is about 24 grams of protein—less than half the government figure. These 24 grams are easily obtainable in meals of properly combined nonanimal food— like a peanut butter sandwich on whole wheat bread, for example, or a plate of pasta or rice with beans.

HEALTH PROBLEMS ASSOCIATED WITH ANIMAL PRODUCTS

Many Americans are in a quandary. On the one hand, they are being told that they should get sufficient protein and that that is possible only if they eat animal products. On the other hand, more and more evidence shows that animal products are responsible for a host of ailments, ranging from constipation and obesity to heart disease and prostate cancer.

Red meat is a particularly bad food for human beings, who were never made to be carnivorous in the first place. Carnivores have an extremely short intestinal tract so that meat passes through quickly. Humans, however, are modeled after vegetarian animals; we have an intestine that measures some twenty-two feet. When we eat meat, it can stay in our intestines for up to three days, during which time it can putrify and poison our whole body. Over time this can lead to prostrate cancer in men, as well as many other ailments. Red meat is also full of saturated fat, cholesterol, antibiotics, and often nitrates, preservatives, and countless other additives. It is *very* high in calories; a twelve-ounce steak contains over a thousand calories.

Milk is high in cholesterol and is not easily digested, which can lead to allergies. It also causes mucous to build up in the body.

The major problem with virtually all animal products on the market today is the high quantities of drug and chemical residues that they contain. Red meats, processed meats, and luncheon meats are all treated with nitrates to preserve their red colors. (Ordinarily they would be gray.) Beef, pork, lamb, and chicken are all heavily treated with antibiotics to stave off infection, which would otherwise run rampant in these animals' unsanitary and overcrowded living conditions.[10] Antibiotics stay in the meat when we consume it. This can make us build up a tolerance to the antibiotics, so that when we really need them, they are of no avail.

Not even fish—unless it is a deep-water fish that is very fresh—is without drawbacks. Mercury and toxic wastes build up in fish that live close to shore, especially in oysters and clams, which filter some twenty gallons of water a day through their bodies. Crustaceans like crabs and lobsters are the scavengers of the sea and can be equally tainted.

Even eggs, the ideal protein, can be tainted by the chemicals and additives in chicken feed and by chemicals added to ensure shell hardness and the correct consistency and color of the yolk.

GETTING CALCIUM FROM HEALTHY SOURCES

Another serious problem with animal-source nutrition is its potential for leading to calcium deficiencies. Although milk is high in calcium, like other animal products it is difficult to digest. It is also high in phosphorus, which binds to calcium, making it unabsorbable; the calcium is then lost in the urine. Hence although the calcium is there, we cannot use it.

Osteoporosis is a disease caused by a calcium deficiency in which the bones lose density and become porous and brittle, causing them to break more easily. It strikes mostly women after the age of forty, crippling many and leaving many with stooped posture.

Recent studies have shown that in countries where few meat or dairy products are consumed, osteoporosis is virtually unknown, while in the five countries consuming the largest amounts of these products, osteoporosis has its highest incidence.[11]

Getting your calcium requirements from a variety of unprocessed natural foods can help prevent osteoporosis and other effects of calcium deficiency. Some good sources are dark leafy vegetables, cauliflower, sesame seeds, soy beans, carob flour, dried fruits, and sea vegetables. You can also get all your calcium requirements from a good supplement. Chelated calcium lactate, calcium citrate, and calcium gluconate are superior choices; bone meal is not as good.

ANOTHER LOOK AT NPU: THE EGG PROJECT

The Egg Project was developed over a period of thirteen years. I undertook the Project because vegetarians were constantly being told that they were not getting enough protein; in fact, many people did not become vegetarian out of fear of becoming sick and malnourished due to insufficient protein. This fear was of course fed massively by the meat- and dairy-producing lobbies, which want all Americans to feel that they literally cannot live without their products.

However, a careful examination of the *scientific* basis for various studies' conclusions about the amounts of protein in foods and protein quality has led me to challenge the entrenched ideas that most Americans hold about protein.

Two specific aspects to the protein myth caught my attention. First, the studies that supposedly determined our protein needs were based on infant rats, not on humans, and on the protein content in rat milk, which is much higher than human milk. It stands to reason that the protein requirements for infant rats, which mature in a matter of weeks, would be much greater than the protein requirements for infant human beings, who mature over a period of years. This fact is reflected in the high protein content of rat milk as opposed to the low protein content in human milk. Nevertheless, these studies have remained unchallenged for years as proof that we need much more protein than we actually do.

The second aspect of the protein myth that caught my attention was that people were being systematically discouraged from eating vegetable protein and being indoctrinated to believe that animal protein was the only *real* source of protein. The theory ran something like this in most nutrition books: If beef is 20 percent protein and I eat a 16-ounce steak, then I am getting 20 percent of that 16-ounce steak in protein that my body can use (or close to 90 grams of protein).*

---

*(Twenty percent of 16 ounces is 3.2 ounces. There are 28 grams in 1 ounce; hence I get 89.6 grams of protein.)

So, the theory goes, I should eat lots of beef, milk, eggs, and fish to make sure I am getting enough protein and to make sure that these high-protein foods are the only good source of protein.

This reasoning is not only misleading; it can also be harmful to your health. Nutritional experts now agree that the egg has the protein that is most fully utilized by our bodies. It is not the highest in protein; but the protein it has is 95 percent utilized by our bodies. This is not the case for other animal products, which have a substantially lower NPU. Here are the NPUs for the most common protein products:

Eggs:	94	Cheese:	70
Milk:	82	Meat and poultry:	67
Fish:	80	Tofu (soybean curd):	65

This means that in addition to being difficult to digest and high in calories and saturated fats, only 67 percent of the protein in meat can actually be utilized by the body. Viewed in this light, meat may not be such a great source of protein after all.[12]

Another problem with the traditional protein theories is that they had many people eating much more protein than they needed. Because of this protein-deficiency phobia, many Americans eat eggs with bacon or sausage and milk for breakfast, a hamburger or cheeseburger for lunch, and a nice big juicy steak for dinner. Despite the poor absorption of the protein in most of these animal foods, people on these kinds of diets were often getting over 200 grams of protein, when at the most they need between 40 and 60 grams per day. As I mentioned earlier, just this excess protein (not to count the fat, calories, and burden on digestion) can cause kidney and liver damage and send toxins throughout the body, due to the urea released as a by-product of protein metabolism.

To summarize:
1. We are getting too much protein.
2. We are generally allergic to the protein we eat.
3. This excess protein is directly responsible for breast and prostate cancer as well as for kidney and liver damage.
4. Not all the protein that we eat is high-quality, well-utilized protein.

To resolve these problems and provide a reliable way for vegetarians and people interested in improving their diet, I undertook the Egg Project. Basically the Project entailed seeing the egg as a model for ideal protein utilization and using the egg's amino acid distribution as a model against which other foods were compared.

With the assistance of Hillard Fitzky, Ph.D., a brilliant computer programmer, I began to compare various foods with the egg to determine their quality of protein. Among the various animal foods I found that their amino acid distribution not only did not match but often was not even close to that of the egg. This meant that although these products had a high protein content, much of it was not protein that we could use; it was not a "high-quality" protein.

However, when I compared one-hundred commonly eaten vegetarian foods with the egg, I found something surprising. Contrary to the myth that these foods are "low-quality" proteins, capable of sustaining but not promoting life, I found that they contain all nine of the essential amino acids and that without even combining many of them they had protein that was more readily utilized than that of many of the animal products; that is, their protein more closely matched the amino acid distribution of the egg.

THE LIMITING AMINO ACID   When you eat protein, all the essential amino acids must be present in the blood at the site of the cell in the right proportions in order for that protein to be utilized by the body. The extent to which a particular amino acid is lacking or is available only in short supply will determine how much of a protein can be used at that moment. For example, if beef is low in lysine (one of the essential amino acids), then the protein in beef can be utilized only to the extent that lysine is present.[13]

THE VEGETARIAN ALTERNATIVE   Using the egg as the model to duplicate as closely as possible, I compared the amino acid content of around a hundred commonly used vegetarian foods in various combinations of twos and threes. The computer compared their amino acids with those of the egg to come up with a higher quality food. Once the computer started to print out, it printed more than a million combinations. The ones I was interested in were those having higher amounts of usable protein than any animal protein (except, of course, the egg). These combinations are listed in the table at the end of this book; they form the basis for the recipes in Chapter 8. All the recipes have been selected on the basis of their high quality of usable protein.

We always have a pool of amino acids in our bloodstream (except when we get up in the morning), from which we can draw to compensate for a limiting amino acid. By eating a highly diverse diet, amino acids from various foods will compensate for the limiting amino acid in another food you may eat. This compensatory effect is less likely to occur when you eat a variety of foods.

The advantage that the Egg Project technique has over other food combining techniques is it shows you exactly which foods to combine and what amount of protein—high quality, utilizable protein—you will be getting.

THE RECIPES

These vegetarian recipes in Chapter 8 exclude preservatives, additives, caffeine, and sugar. They are divided into a four-day rotational plan so that no single food is eaten more than once every four days. Zucchini, for example, is an ingredient on day one, so it does not appear on any other day.

Following a rotational diet, as we have discussed, is a good way to prevent new allergies and to handle existing sensitivities.

If you are allergic to a specific food in any recipe, do not use that recipe!

Fortunately, it isn't necessary to learn the amounts and proportions of essential amino acids in various foods in order to eat properly. In the appendix are listed thousands of combinations of healthy foods from which to choose.

Luckily for all of us, the healthiest combinations also seem to be the best tasting.

Bon appetit!

CHAPTER EIGHT

Recipes

When choosing a recipe for a particular day, be sure to keep the ingredients consistent. You may substitute your "vegetable of the day" in any of the recipes.

Caroby Coconut Bulgur

6 ounces bulgur
1½ ounces coconut, shredded and
    unsweetened
1½ ounces cashews, chopped
1 tablespoon carob powder

Cook bulgur in a medium pot with 15 ounces water. **Bring** to a boil, then lower heat. **Cook** until water is absorbed. **Add** remaining ingredients and mix well.

Serves 1.

Peachy Coconut Bulgur

6 ounces bulgur
1½ ounces coconut, shredded and
    unsweetened
1½ ounces cashews, chopped
1½ ounces dried peaches, chopped
1 teaspoon cinnamon

Pour bulgur into a medium mixing bowl. **Soak** in 15 ounces hot water, with cover, for approximately 12 minutes, or until water has been absorbed by the bulgur. **Add** coconut, cashews, peaches, and cinnamon. **Combine** all the ingredients.

Serves 1.

Cinnamon Cashew Bulgur

6 ounces bulgur
1½ ounces coconut, shredded and
    unsweetened
1½ ounces cashews, chopped
1½ ounces sunflower seeds
1 ounce dried nectarines
1 teaspoon cinnamon

Cook bulgur in a medium pot with 15 ounces water. **Bring** to a boil, then lower heat. Cooking time is approximately 12 minutes. **Add** remaining ingredients and mix well.
Serves 1.

Tasty Split-Pea Melange

3 ounces bulgur
3 ounces split peas
3 ounces watercress, chopped
3 ounces red cabbage, sliced and
    chopped
1½ ounces coconut, shredded and
    unsweetened
1 teaspoon minced garlic
½ teaspoon coriander
½ teaspoon salt

Pour bulgur into a bowl with 10 ounces hot water, covered. **Soak** until all water is absorbed, about 15 minutes. **Pour** split peas into a saucepan with 12 ounces water. **Allow** to cook over medium heat for about 35 minutes. **Add** watercress and cabbage. **Mix** well. **Combine** remaining ingredients with bulgur/split-pea mixture. **Mix** again. **Serve** at room temperature.
Serves 2.

Hearty Noodle Soup

6 ounces buckwheat noodles
6 ounces carrots, sliced into bite-
    size pieces
6 ounces mushrooms, sliced into
    bite-size pieces
6 ounces broccoli, cut into
    flowerettes

Drop noodles into a medium saucepan with salted boiling water. **Cook** for 5 minutes. **Set** aside. **Place** vegetables in a medium saucepan with 4 cups boiling water. **Add** rosemary, salt, bay leaf, and oil, and cook over medium-high heat for 10 minutes. **Put**

4 cups water
½ teaspoon rosemary
¾ teaspoon salt
1 bay leaf
3 tablespoons sunflower oil

half this mixture into a blender, and purée until well blended. **Return** purée to soup. **Add** noodles, and cook for another 8 minutes.

Yields 4 to 5 cups.

Split Pea Veggie Soup

6 ounces split peas
6 ounces bulgur
6 ounces cauliflower, cut into flowerettes
3 ounces onion, chopped
3 ounces carrots, chopped
3 tablespoons sunflower oil
1 teaspoon minced garlic
½ teaspoon salt

Cook split peas in a medium saucepan with enough water to cover. **Bring** to a boil, lower heat and cook for 15 minutes. **Cook** bulgur in saucepan with 15 ounces water. **Bring** to boil and lower heat. **Combine** all ingredients together and cook for additional 15 minutes over low heat.

Yields 4 to 5 cups approximately

Grandma's Kidney Bean Soup

6 ounces kidney beans
6 ounces bulgur
1½ ounces celery, chopped
1½ ounces carrots, sliced
1½ ounces onions, chopped
½ teaspoon minced garlic
½ teaspoon cumin

Soak beans overnight in 3 cups water. In the morning, rinse the beans and add 4 cups fresh water. **Transfer** to medium pot and cover. **Bring** to a boil and lower to medium heat. **Cook** bulgur in 15 ounces water in medium saucepan. **Bring** to a boil and lower to medium heat. When beans have been cooking for 1½ hours, add bulgur and remaining ingredients. **Cook** for additional 15 minutes. **Place** half of this mixture in blender and puree for 15 seconds. **Add** back to the rest of the soup.

Yields 4 to 5 cups approximately

Corianut Bulgur Casserole

3 ounces bulgur
1½ ounces peanut butter
½ teaspoon coriander
½ teaspoon minced garlic
½ teaspoon tamari
1½ tablespoons sunflower oil
1½ ounces sweet onions, chopped
    finely
1 ounce green peppers, chopped
    finely

Preheat oven to 325 degrees. Lightly grease with sunflower oil a 5 × 7 baking dish with cover. **Cook** bulgur in a medium pot in 12 ounces water. **Bring** to a boil then lower heat. Cooking time is approximately 20 minutes. **Set** aside. **Combine** peanut butter with coriander, garlic, tamari, oil and 2 ounces water in a blender. **Blend** until smooth. **Saute** onions and peppers in sunflower oil. **Combine** with the bulgur. **Pour** peanut butter mixture into bulgur and mix well. **Transfer** to baking dish, cover and bake for 20 minutes.

Serves 1.

Thai Squash

1 (3 ounces) butternut squash
1½ ounces scallions, chopped
1½ ounces peanuts
2 tablespoons sunflower oil
½ teaspoon salt
½ teaspoon fresh parsley, chopped
1 teaspoon minced garlic
3 ounces avocado, sliced

Preheat oven to 400 degrees Fahrenheit. Lightly grease a 4 × 8-inch baking pan with sunflower oil. **Cut** squash in half. **Remove** seeds and discard them. **Place** squash cut-side down in a baking dish with ⅓ inch water. **Bake** for 40 minutes. When squash is cool enough to handle, remove the skin and chop into 1-inch pieces. **Lower** heat in oven to 350 degrees. **Place** scallions, peanuts, oil, salt, parsley, and garlic in blender. **Purée** until sauce consistency is achieved. **Place** squash into baking pan, and pour sauce on top. **Cover** and bake at 350 degrees for 20 minutes. Upon serving, place avocado slices on top as garnish.

Serves 2.

Summer Picnic Salad

3 ounces bulgur
3 ounces broccoli, cut into flowerettes
2 ounces red onion, sliced
3 ounces avocado, cut into bite-size pieces
1 ounce coconut, shredded and unsweetened
1½ ounces sunflower seeds
1 teaspoon oregano
1 teaspoon tamari
2 teaspoons apple cider vinegar
2 tablespoons sunflower oil

Pour bulgur into a medium mixing bowl. **Soak** in 10 ounces hot water, with cover, for approximately 12 minutes, or until water has been absorbed by the bulgur. **Steam** the broccoli for approximately 8 minutes. **Add** broccoli, onion, avocado, and coconut. **Toss** gently so as not to mash avocado. **Add** remaining ingredients, and toss again. **Serve** chilled.

Serves 2.

Buckwheat Noodle Potpourri

6 ounces buckwheat noodles
6 ounces cauliflower, cut into flowerettes and steamed
6 ounces onions, chopped
3 ounces marinated artichoke, chopped
1 teaspoon oregano
½ teaspoon coriander
½ teaspoon salt
3 tablespoons sunflower oil

Drop noodles into medium saucepan with salted boiling water. **Drain** and rinse. **Toss** with remaining ingredients.

Serves 2.

Sweet Mango Kanten

4 ounces mango
12 ounces pineapple-coconut juice
2 heaping tablespoons agar-agar
1 tablespoon date sugar
1 tablespoon raisins
1 teaspoon vanilla
1 ounce coconut, shredded and
　　unsweetened
1 ounce strawberries, halved

Blend mango with pineapple-coconut juice in a saucepan. **Bring** to a boil, then lower heat. **Add** agar-agar and stir until dissolved. **Simmer** for 5 minutes. **Add** date sugar, raisins, and vanilla. **Place** in refrigerator until mixture begins to gel – about 10 minutes. **Drop** in coconut and strawberries. **Chill** for 1 hour.
Serves 2.

DAY TWO

Figgy Cashew Rice

6 ounces brown rice
1½ ounces coconut, shredded and
　　unsweetened
1½ ounces cashews, chopped
1½ ounces figs, chopped
2 ounces pineapple-coconut juice
1½ ounces sunflower seeds

Pour rice into a medium saucepan with 14 ounces water. **Bring** water to a boil, then lower heat and simmer for 30 minutes. **Add** coconut, cashews, and figs. **Mix** thoroughly. **Place** half the mixture into a blender, and purée with pineapple-coconut juice for a few seconds. **Add** puréed mixture back to the rest of the rice. **Sprinkle** sunflower seeds on top.
Serves 1.

Alfalfa Vegetable Rice Salad

3 ounces brown rice
3 ounces carrots, cut into bite-size
　　pieces

Pour rice into a medium saucepan with 12 ounces water. **Bring** water to a boil; then lower heat and allow to

1⅓ ounces onion, chopped medium
    fine
¼ teaspoon fresh parsley, chopped
    fine
1½ ounces cashews, chopped
2 tablespoons sunflower oil
1½ teaspoons cumin
¾ teaspoon salt
3 teaspoons apple cider vinegar
3 ounces alfalfa sprouts

simmer for 30 minutes. **Add** carrots, onion, parsley, and cashews. In a medium skillet, place the sunflower oil. **Sauté** the rice mixture in the oil, adding the cumin and salt. **Remove** from skillet to bowl, and add vinegar and sprouts. **Mix** thoroughly. **Serve** at room temperature.

Serves 1.

Gary's Spinach Salad

3 ounces spinach, torn into bite-size
    pieces
3 ounces red onion, sliced
1½ ounces peanuts
3 ounces marinated artichokes
3 ounces avocado, cut into bite-size
    pieces
½ teaspoon basil
¼ teaspoon black pepper
1½ tablespoons sunflower oil

Combine all ingredients in a medium salad bowl and toss.

Serves 1.

Mama's Stuffed Cabbage

1 head cabbage, steamed
3 ounces brown rice
3 ounces split peas
2 ounces onion, grated
2 ounces mushrooms, sliced
1½ ounces cashews, chopped
2 tablespoons sunflower oil
1 teaspoon minced garlic
½ teaspoon rosemary
1 teaspoon tamari

Preheat oven to 350 degrees Fahrenheit. Lightly grease a 4 × 8-inch casserole dish with 2 tablespoons sunflower oil. **Separate** leaves from steamed cabbage after it has cooled. **Pour** brown rice into medium saucepan with 12 ounces water. **Bring** to a boil, then lower heat and simmer for 30 minutes. **Do** likewise with split peas. **Set** aside. **Combine** all the remaining ingredients with the brown rice and split peas. **Mix** thoroughly. **Arrange** 1 to 2 tablespoons of mixture on each leaf, depending on size of cabbage leaf. **Fold** like an envelope. **Place** in casserole dish and cover. **Bake** for 20 minutes or until thoroughly heated.

Serves 2 to 4.

Simple Rice and Bean Casserole

3 ounces kidney beans
3 ounces brown rice
1½ ounces cashew pieces
1½ ounces filberts, finely chopped
2 tablespoons sunflower oil
1 tablespoon mustard
¼ teaspoon cayenne
½ teaspoon salt

Lightly oil a 4 × 8-inch baking dish with sunflower oil. **Preheat** oven to 375 degrees Fahrenheit. **Soak** beans overnight in a bowl with 16 ounces water. In the morning, rinse the beans, transfer to a medium saucepan, and add 16 ounces fresh water. **Bring** to a boil, and then cook over medium heat for 1½ to 1¾ hours.

Pour rice into a medium saucepan with 12 ounces water. **Bring** to a boil, lower heat, and simmer for 35 minutes.

Place cashews and filberts into a blender; add 2 ounces water as well as oil, mustard, cayenne, and salt. **Purée** until mixture achieves a sauce consistency.

Transfer beans and rice into baking dish. **Pour** sauce on top. **Bake** at 375 degrees for 15 minutes.

Serves 2.

Split-Pea Vegetable Bake

3 ounces split peas
3 ounces eggplant
3 ounces broccoli, cut into
   flowerettes
3 ounces mushrooms, sliced
1 ounce onion, chopped finely
3 ounces cashews, chopped
1 teaspoon minced garlic
½ teaspoon oregano
¼ teaspoon basil
½ teaspoon salt
2 tablespoons sunflower oil

Lightly grease a 4 × 8-inch baking pan with sunflower oil. **Preheat** oven to 350 degrees Fahrenheit. **Pour** split peas into a medium saucepan with 12 ounces water. **Set** over medium heat for approximately 35 minutes. **Steam** the broccoli and mushrooms for 5 minutes. **Place** split peas into a blender with 2 ounces water, onion, cashews, garlic, oregano, basil, salt, and oil. **Purée** until mixture achieves a sauce consistency. **Place** eggplant in baking pan; add broccoli and mushrooms. **Pour** split-pea sauce on top. Bake for 20 minutes.

Serves 2.

Delectable Brown Rice Pudding

3 ounces brown rice
6 ounces mango
1½ ounces coconut, shredded and
   unsweetened
1½ ounces figs
10 ounces pineapple-coconut juice
2 heaping teaspoons Ener-G-Egg
   Replacer

To cook rice, pour in a saucepan with 8 to 10 ounces water. **Bring** to a boil, then lower heat. **Simmer** for 20 to 25 minutes. **Place** all ingredients in a blender. **Purée** until smooth. **Cook** in saucepan over medium heat for 5 minutes, stirring frequently. **Chill** for 45 minutes.

Yields approximately 15 ounces.

Brown Rice Broccoli Burgers

3 ounces split peas
3 ounces brown rice
3 ounces broccoli, cut into
    flowerettes
1½ ounces onions, sautéed
2 ounces cashews
4 tablespoons sunflower oil
2 heaping teaspoons arrowroot
1 teaspoon coriander
1 teaspoon salt

Lightly grease a baking sheet with sunflower oil. **Preheat** oven to 350 degrees Fahrenheit. **Pour** split peas into a medium saucepan with 12 ounces water. **Set** over medium heat for approximately 35 minutes.

Pour rice into a medium saucepan with 12 ounces water. **Bring** to a boil, lower heat, and allow to simmer for 35 minutes.

Place all ingredients into a blender, and blend until mixture is coarsely ground. **Transfer** to bowl and mix thoroughly. **Form** patties with the mixture and place on baking sheet. **Bake** for 30 minutes or until crispy on outside.

Serves 2.

Kidney Kale Burgers

3 ounces kidney beans
3 ounces kale, steamed
1½ ounces onions, sautéed
2 ounces tomato sauce
3 tablespoons sunflower oil
2 heaping teaspoons arrowroot
1 teaspoon salt
½ teaspoon oregano

Preheat oven to 350 degrees Fahrenheit. Lightly grease a baking sheet with sunflower oil. **Soak** kidney beans overnight in 16 ounces water. In the morning, rinse the beans, transfer to a medium saucepan, and add 16 ounces fresh water. **Cook** for 1½ to 1¾ hours over medium heat. **Place** all ingredients in a blender until mixture is coarsely ground. **Make** patties from the mixture, and place on baking sheet. **Bake** for 30 minutes or until crispy on the outside.

Serves 2.

Brown Rice Kasha Burger

3 ounces brown rice

1½ ounces buckwheat groats (kasha)

2 ounces filberts, chopped finely

3 ounces carrots

3 heaping teaspoons Ener-G-Egg Replacer

2 tablespoons sunflower oil

1 tablespoon fresh dill, finely chopped

1 teaspoon minced garlic

½ teaspoon salt

Preheat oven to 350 degrees Fahrenheit. Lightly grease a baking sheet with sunflower oil. **Pour** rice into a medium saucepan with 12 ounces water. **Bring** to boil, lower heat, and allow to simmer for 35 minutes.

Pour buckwheat into 6 ounces water in a small saucepan. **Bring** to boil, lower heat, and simmer for 25 minutes.

Place all ingredients into a blender, and blend until coarsely ground. **Transfer** to a bowl and mix well. **Form** patties about 2 inches in diameter and place on baking sheet. **Put** in oven to bake for 25 minutes or until crispy on the outside.

Yields 6 burgers.

Indian Sun Rice Burgers

3 ounces brown rice

2 ounces sunflower seeds

1½ ounces brown rice flour

3 tablespoons chopped scallions

2 tablespoons sunflower oil

2 heaping teaspoons Ener-G-Egg Replacer

2 teaspoons tamari

1 teaspoon minced garlic

½ teaspoon cumin

Preheat oven to 350 degrees Fahrenheit. Lightly grease a baking sheet with sunflower oil. **Pour** rice into a medium saucepan with 12 ounces water. **Bring** to a boil, lower heat, and allow to simmer for 35 minutes.

Put rice and sunflower seeds in a blender. **Purée.** If necessary, turn blender off and press mixture down with a wooden spoon (be sure blade has stopped moving), then resume blending. You may have to do this a few times. The final mixture will be sticky. **Transfer** to a mixing bowl. **Add** brown rice flour and remaining ingredients. **Form** into patties 2 inches or so in diameter. **Place** on baking sheet for 25 minutes or until crispy on outside.

Yields 4 burgers.

Peppery Kidney Bean Soup

3 ounces kidney beans
6 ounces broccoli, chopped into bite-size flowerettes
3 ounces red pepper, chopped medium fine
3 ounces green pepper, chopped medium fine
1 teaspoon onion, minced
½ teaspoon black pepper
½ teaspoon salt
3 tablespoons sunflower oil

Soak beans in a bowl overnight in 3 cups water. In the morning, rinse the beans, transfer to a medium saucepan, and add 4 cups water. **Bring** beans to a boil, then lower to medium heat. **Keep** the cover on. In a separate bowl, combine remaining ingredients and toss. After beans have cooked for 1½ hours, add vegetable mixture to beans. **Place** half this mixture into a blender, and purée for 15 seconds. **Return** to soup and mix well.

Yields 4 to 5 cups.

Kinky Kidney Bean Soup

3 ounces kidney beans
6 ounces brown rice
1½ ounces cashew pieces
½ teaspoon coriander
½ teaspoon cumin
¾ teaspoon salt
3 tablespoons sunflower oil

Soak beans overnight in a bowl with 3 cups water. In the morning, rinse the beans, transfer to a medium saucepan, and add 4 cups water. **Bring** beans to a boil, and then lower to medium heat. **Cook** with cover. To cook rice, pour it into a medium saucepan with 12 to 14 ounces water.

Bring the water to a boil, stir once, and lower heat to medium while covered with a lid. **Simmer** slowly until all water is absorbed by rice. After 1½ hours, add rice and other ingredients to the beans. **Cook** for an additional 15 minutes. **Pour** half the mixture into a blender and purée for 15 seconds. **Add** back to the soup and mix well. Yields 4 to 5 cups.

Quick Asparagus Dip

2 ounces brown rice
3 ounces asparagus
2 ounces onion, sliced
4 tablespoons sunflower oil
1 teaspoon salt
2 teaspoons mustard
4 tablespoons cider vinegar
3 ounces water

To cook rice, pour into a small saucepan with 5 or 6 ounces water. **Bring** to a boil, then lower heat. **Simmer** for about 20 to 25 minutes. **Steam** or blanch asparagus until tender, then run immediately under cold water to preserve fresh green color. **Chop** crudely and purée in blender with rice and all other ingredients.

Yields approximately 12 ounces.

Asparagus Mushroom Dip

2 ounces brown rice
3 ounces asparagus
2 ounces mushrooms, chopped
3 ounces marinated artichokes
4 tablespoons sunflower oil
1 teaspoon minced garlic
½ teaspoon salt
2 tablespoons cider vinegar

To cook rice, pour into a small saucepan with 5 or 6 ounces water. **Bring** to a boil, then lower heat. **Simmer** for about 20 to 25 minutes. **Steam** or blanch asparagus until tender, then run immediately under cold water to preserve fresh green color. **Chop** crudely and purée in blender with rice and all other ingredients.

Yields approximately 9 ounces.

Italian Avocado Dip

1½ ounces brown rice
3 ounces eggplant, sliced
6 ounces avocado, chopped
1 teaspoon minced garlic
½ teaspoon oregano
½ teaspoon salt
3 tablespoons cider vinegar
3 tablespoons sunflower oil

To cook rice, pour into a small saucepan with 4 or 5 ounces water. **Bring** to a boil, then lower heat. **Simmer** for 20 to 25 minutes. **Steam** eggplant until tender. **Purée** in a blender with rice and all other ingredients.

Yields approximately 11 ounces.

DAY 3

Apricot Almond Millet

6 ounces millet
1½ ounces almonds, blanched and chopped
1 ounce dried apricots
1½ ounces brewer's yeast

Cook millet in 13 ounces water. When water comes to boil, lower heat. **Stir** occasionally. **Cook** 30 minutes. **Add** remaining ingredients to millet. **Mix** well.

Serves 1.

Banana Cream of Wheat

6 ounces cream of wheat
1 banana, mashed
½ tablespoon maple syrup
1½ ounces brewer's yeast

Cook cream of wheat in 12 ounces water over medium heat for 10 minutes or until done, stirring occasionally. **Add** all other ingredients. Mix well.

Serves 1.

Aduki Zucchini Salad

3 ounces aduki beans
3 ounces zucchini, sliced
3 ounces red pepper, chopped
1 ounce onion, finely chopped
2 tablespoons olive oil
½ teaspoon fresh parsley, finely chopped
½ teaspoon rosemary
½ teaspoon salt

Soak beans overnight in 16 ounces water. In the morning, rinse the beans, transfer to a saucepan, and replace with 16 ounces fresh water. **Cook** over medium heat for 1 to 1½ hours. **Steam** zucchini. **Toss** together with all other ingredients.
Serves 1.

Summer Potato Salad

3 ounces potato
3 ounces onion, chopped
3 ounces mushrooms, chopped
1½ ounces triticale flour
1½ ounces tahini
1½ ounces toasted sesame seeds
½ teaspoon salt
2 tablespoons sesame oil
1 ounce fresh parsley, chopped

Bake potato for 40 minutes at 400 degrees Fahrenheit, or until a fork easily pierces it. When cooled, cut into ½-inch cubes. **Blend** onions and mushrooms in a medium bowl. **Add** triticale flour, tahini, sesame seeds, salt, and 2 ounces water. **Sauté** potatoes and all other ingredients in a skillet with sesame oil for 4 minutes over medium heat. **Add** parsley.
Serves 2.

Variety Veggie Salad

3 ounces spinach
3 ounces red pepper, chopped
3 ounces okra, cut in half
3 ounces yellow squash, sliced
1½ ounces triticale flour
1 teaspoon minced onion

Steam spinach, pepper, okra, and yellow squash for about 8 minutes. **Combine** triticale flour with 2 ounces water, onion, salt, garlic, and oregano. In a skillet sauté vegetables with triticale sauce for 3 minutes in sesame

1 teaspoon salt

½ teaspoon minced garlic

½ teaspoon oregano

2 tablespoons sesame oil

1½ ounces almonds, blanched and
slivered.

oil. **Sprinkle** with almonds.
Serves 3.

Gary's Primavera

3 ounces dry spaghetti

6 ounces tomato, finely chopped

1½ ounces minced scallions

1½ ounces sliced mushrooms

½ teaspoon cumin

½ teaspoon rosemary

½ teaspoon minced garlic

½ teaspoon salt

2 tablespoon olive oil

1½ ounces pumpkin seeds

Cook spaghetti in 24 ounces water
for 10 minutes or until done to your
taste. **Sauté** tomato, scallions, and
mushrooms in a skillet with herbs,
salt, and oil over low heat for 15
minutes. **Drain,** and toss the spaghetti with the pumpkin seeds and sautéed
vegetables. **Serve** hot.
Serves 1.

Mushroom Sauté

1½ ounces triticale flour

½ teaspoon oregano

½ teaspoon basil

¼ teaspoon tarragon

½ teaspoon tamari

¼ teaspoon salt

1 tablespoon sesame oil

6 ounces mushrooms, sliced

3 ounces zucchini, cut into bite-size
pieces

1½ ounces onions, sliced

Preheat oven to 325 degrees
Fahrenheit. Lightly oil a 4 × 8-inch
baking dish with sesame oil. In a mixing bowl, combine triticale flour with
2 ounces water, oregano, basil, tarragon, tamari, salt, and oil. While
quickly stir-frying vegetables, gradually incorporate triticale sauce. **Sauté**
4 minutes. **Transfer** ingredients to
baking dish. Cover and bake for 20
minutes.
Serves 2.

Aduki Potato Casserole

3 ounces aduki beans
3 ounces millet
3 ounces potato
3 ounces spinach, torn into bite-size
  pieces
1½ ounces onion, sliced
2 tablespoons olive oil
½ teaspoon basil
½ teaspoon salt
1 teaspoon apple cider vinegar
¼ teaspoon paprika
1 teaspoon fresh parsley, finely
  chopped

Preheat oven to 400 degrees Fahrenheit. Lightly grease a 4 × 8″ baking pan with sesame oil. **Soak** beans overnight in 16 ounces water. In the morning, rinse the beans, transfer to a saucepan, and replace with 16 ounces fresh water. Beans should cook over medium heat for 1 to 1½ hours. **Pour** millet into 12 ounces water in a medium saucepan. **Set** over medium heat for 25 minutes. **Place** potato in oven, and bake for 40 minutes. When cooled, cut potato in ½-inch pieces. **Lower** oven temperature to 350 degrees. **Sauté** spinach and onion in a skillet with olive oil. **Add** basil, salt, and vinegar. **Sauté** for 3 minutes. **Combine** all ingredients in a mixing bowl and toss. **Transfer** to baking pan, cover, and place in oven for 20 minutes.

Serves 2.

Asparagus Bean Casserole

3 ounces aduki beans
3 ounces millet
3 ounces asparagus, cut into bite-
  size pieces
3 ounces mushrooms, sliced
3 ounces pumpkin seeds
2 tablespoons sesame oil
½ teaspoon oregano
½ teaspoon salt

Preheat oven to 375 degrees Fahrenheit. Lightly grease a baking pan with sesame oil. **Soak** beans overnight in 16 ounces water. In the morning, rinse the beans, transfer to a saucepan, and add 16 ounces fresh water. **Set** over medium heat for 1 to 1½ hours.

Pour millet into 12 ounces water.

Set over medium heat for 25 minutes. Steam asparagus and mushrooms. Combine all ingredients in a mixing bowl and toss. Transfer to baking pan and bake for 15 minuts.

Serves 1.

Carrot Millet Patties

3 ounces millet
1½ ounces spanish onion, chopped
2 ounces carrots, sliced
2 ounces pumpkin seeds
3 tablespoons olive oil
1 teaspoon minced garlic
½ teaspoon coriander
2 heaping teaspoons arrowroot

Preheat oven to 350 degrees Fahrenheit. Lightly grease a baking sheet with sesame oil. Pour millet into to 12 ounces water. Set over medium heat, and cook for 25 minutes. Steam onion and carrots. Place all ingredients in a blender until coarsely ground. Transfer to a mixing bowl and mix well. Form patties 1 to 2 inches in diameter, and place on baking sheet. Bake for 30 minutes or until crispy on outside.

Serves 2.

Broccoli Potato Patties

3 ounces potato, sliced ¼ inch thick
3 ounces wheat flakes
1½ ounces broccoli, cut into
  flowerettes
1½ ounces chives, chopped
1 ounce sesame seeds
4 tablespoons olive oil
2 heaping teaspoons Ener-G-Egg
  Replacer
1 teaspoon minced garlic

Preheat oven to 350 degrees Fahrenheit. Lightly grease a baking sheet with sesame oil. Boil potato until done, and cube. Pour wheat flakes into a saucepan with 8 ounces water. Bring to a boil, and lower heat. Steam broccoli until tender. Place all ingredients into a blender, and purée until coarsely ground. Transfer to a mixing bowl. Form patties approx-

½ teaspoon oregano
½ teaspoon salt

imately 1 to 2 inches in diameter. **Place** patties onto baking sheet, and bake for 30 minutes or until crispy on the outside.

Serves 2.

Curried Aduki Burgers

3 ounces aduki beans
1½ ounces onions, sliced
1 ounce carrots, sliced
2 ounces sesame seeds
2 heaping teaspoons Ener-G-Egg
   Replacer
2 tablespoons olive oil
1 teaspoon curry
½ teaspoon salt

Preheat oven to 350 degrees Fahrenheit. Lightly grease a baking sheet with sesame oil. **Soak** beans overnight in 16 ounces water. In the morning, rinse the beans, transfer to a saucepan, and add 16 ounces fresh water. Beans should cook over medium heat for 1 to 1½ hours. **Sauté** onion and carrots. **Put** all ingredients together into a blender, and purée until completely ground. **Form** into patties approximately 1 to 2 inches in diameter. **Place** on baking sheet, and bake for 30 minutes.

Yields 4 burgers.

Mexican Bean Burger

3 ounces aduki beans
3 ounces wheat flakes
2 ounces tomato
2 ounces mushrooms, sliced
2 heaping teaspoons Ener-G-Egg
   Replacer
2 tablespoons olive oil
1 teaspoon minced garlic
½ teaspoon salt

Preheat oven to 350 degrees Fahrenheit. Lightly grease a baking sheet with sesame oil. **Soak** beans overnight in 16 ounces water. In the morning, rinse the beans, transfer to a saucepan, and add 16 ounces fresh water. Beans should cook over medium heat for 1 to 1½ hours. **Pour** wheat flakes into a saucepan with 8 ounces water. **Bring** to a boil, and lower heat. **Combine** all ingredients in a blender, and purée until completely blended. **Form** patties 1 to 2 inches in diameter, and place on baking sheet. **Bake** in oven for 30 minutes or until crispy on outside.

Yields 4 burgers.

Potato Chowder Deluxe

9 ounces potato, sliced
3 tablespoons sesame oil
½ teaspoon cayenne
½ teaspoon salt
3 ounces corn (fresh off the husk or frozen)
6 ounces chopped red pepper

Boil potatoes in a medium saucepan with 4 cups water for 15 minutes. **Place** potato, cooking water, oil, cayenne, and salt in a blender. **Purée. Transfer** back into saucepan, and place back on stove over low heat. **Add** corn and red pepper. **Cook** for 10 to 15 minutes.

Yields 4 to 5 cups.

Okra Cabbage Soup

6 ounces okra
3 ounces chopped red cabbage
3 ounces celery, sliced
3 ounces chopped scallions
1 teaspoon minced garlic
1 teaspoon minced onion
½ teaspoon caraway seeds
½ teaspoon salt

Drop okra into 4 cups salted boiling water, and allow to cook for 10 minutes. **Purée** this soup base in a blender. **Place** back on stove over low heat, and add all remaining ingredients. **Raise** heat to medium, and simmer for 12 minutes.

Yields 4 to 5 cups.

Crunchy Millet Almond Dip

3 ounces millet
1 ounce onion, sliced

Pour millet into a saucepan with 8 to 10 ounces water. **Bring** to a boil,

1½ ounces almond butter
3 tablespoons sesame oil
2 ounces water
½ ounce sesame seeds
1 teaspoon coriander

and lower to medium heat. **Cook** for approximately 20 minutes. **Sauté** onion with small amount sesame oil. **Combine** almond butter with remaining sesame oil and water. **Place** all ingredients in blender, and purée until smooth.

Yields approximately 9 ounces.

Tomato Potato Dip

3 ounces potato, sliced
1½ ounces pumpkin seeds
1½ ounces fresh parsley, chopped
4 tablespoons olive oil
1 teaspoon tomato paste
2 tablespoons cider vinegar
½ teaspoon oregano
½ teaspoon salt

Boil potato in a small saucepan for 15 minutes in 2 to 2½ cups water. **Place** all ingredients into a blender. **Purée** until smooth.

Yields 12 ounces.

Gary's Bean Dip

3 ounces aduki beans
3 ounces potato, sliced
1 ounce celery, finely chopped
1 ounce carrots, finely chopped
1 teaspoon minced onion
½ teaspoon tamari
½ teaspoon cider vinegar
½ teaspoon salt

Soak beans overnight in 16 ounces water. In the morning, rinse, transfer to a saucepan, and add 16 ounces fresh water. Beans should be cooked over medium heat for 1½ hours. **Boil** potato in a small saucepan for 15 minutes in 2 to 2½ cups water. **Place** all ingredients in a blender, and purée until smooth.

Yields 12 ounces.

Apple Berry Kanten

10 ounces apple strawberry juice
2 heaping teaspoons agar-agar

Pour juice into a saucepan, and bring to a boil. **Lower** heat, and add

3 tablespoons maple syrup
2 ounces raspberries
2 ounces blueberries

agar-agar. **Stir** and dissolve agar. **Simmer** for 5 minutes. **Add** maple syrup. **Place** in refrigerator until juice begins to gel, around 10 minutes. **Drop** in berries. **Chill** for 1 hour.

Serves 2.

Melon Peach Pudding

5 ounces melon (cantaloupe, honeydew, cranshaw, etc.)
6 ounces peaches, pitted
6 ounces apple-pineapple juice
4 tablespoons maple syrup
2 heaping teaspoons Ener-G-Egg Replacer
1½ ounces almonds, chopped
Pinch cinnamon

Place all ingredients, except almonds and cinnamon, into a blender. **Purée** until smooth. **Transfer** to a saucepan, and heat for 5 minutes, stirring constantly over medium heat. **Chill** for 45 minutes. **Sprinkle** with almonds and cinnamon.

Serves 2.

DAY 4

Vanilla Soy Malt

8 ounces unsweetened soy milk
2 tablespoons barley malt
½ teaspoon vanilla
Pinch cinnamon

Place all ingredients into a blender, and blend for 2 minutes until frothy.

Serves 1.

Fresh Fruit Barley

6 ounces barley
3 ounces your favorite fruit
1½ ounce walnuts, chopped
2 tablespoons barley malt

In a medium saucepan, cook barley in 14 ounces water for 20 minutes. **Stir** in remaining ingredients.

Serves 1.

Mucho Veggie Salad

3 ounces soy beans
3 ounces broccoli, cut into
    flowerettes
3 ounces red pepper, chopped
3 ounces celery, chopped
1½ tablespoons soy oil
1 teaspoon minced garlic
½ teaspoon chopped dill
½ teaspoon salt
1½ ounces brazil nuts

Soak beans overnight in 16 ounces water. In the morning, rinse the beans, transfer to a saucepan, and add 16 ounces fresh water. **Set** over medium heat for approximately 2 hours. **Steam** broccoli, red pepper, and celery for 8 minutes, or until done to your taste. (Tastes really good when crunchy.)

Combine beans and vegetables. **Add** oil, garlic, dill, and salt. **Toss** in brazil nuts. **Mix** well.

Serves 2.

Tangy Barley Bean Salad

3 ounces chick peas
3 ounces barley
3 ounces okra, cut in half
3 ounces watercress, torn into bite-
    size pieces
2 tablespoons soy oil
2 tablespoons chopped parsley
1 teaspoon minced onion
Juice of ½ lime
½ teaspoon salt

Soak chick peas overnight in 16 ounces water. In the morning, rinse the beans, transfer to a saucepan, and add 20 ounces fresh water. **Cook** for 2 hours or until tender. To cook barley, pour into 16 ounces water. **Bring** to a boil, then lower to medium heat and cook for 25 minutes. **Steam** okra. **Combine** all ingredients together, and mix well.

Serves 2.

Sassy Vegetable Mix

3 ounces snap green beans, cut into
    bite-size pieces
3 ounces brussels sprouts, cut into

Steam beans, brussels sprouts, and cauliflower until tender, for approximately 10 minutes. **Combine** beans,

bite-size flowerettes
3 ounces cauliflower, cut into bite-
    size flowerettes
1½ ounces walnuts
2 tablespoons soy oil
1 teaspoon minced garlic
½ teaspoon basil
½ teaspoon tarragon
¼ teaspoon black pepper

walnuts, and remaining ingredients with 2 ounces water in a blender. **Purée** until smooth. **Pour** sauce over brussels sprouts and cauliflower. **Serve** hot or cold.

Serves 2.

Gary's Black Bean Salad

3 ounces black beans
3 ounces carrots, sliced
3 ounces zucchini, sliced
1½ ounces brazil nuts, finely
    chopped
2 tablespoons corn oil
1 tablespoon minced onion
½ teaspoon salt
½ teaspoon oregano

Soak beans overnight in 16 ounces water. In the morning, rinse the beans, transfer to a saucepan, and add 16 ounces fresh water. **Cook** over medium heat for 1½ hours. **Steam** carrots and zucchini for approximately 8 minutes, or until done to your taste. **Combine** all ingredients, mixing well. **Serve** at room temperature.

Serves 2.

Brazilian Beans and Vegetable Delight

3 ounces lima beans
3 ounces snap green beans, cut into
    bite-size pieces
3 ounces tofu, cut into ½-inch
    cubes
3 ounces yellow squash, sliced into
    bite-size pieces
1½ ounces brazil nuts
2 tablespoons soy oil

Preheat oven to 350 degrees Fahrenheit. Lightly grease a 4 x 8″ baking dish with soy oil. **Soak** beans overnight in 16 ounces water. In the morning, rinse the beans, transfer to a medium saucepan, and add 16 ounces fresh water. **Set** over medium heat for 1½ hours.

Combine all ingredients, mixing

1 tablespoon honey
1 teaspoon minced garlic
½ teaspoon coriander

well. Transfer to baking dish, cover, and bake for 20 minutes.

Serves 2.

Indonesian Tempeh

3 ounces chick peas
½ ounce dulse, dry
3 ounces tempeh, cut into ½-inch cubes
3 ounces mushrooms, sliced
3 ounces soy sprouts
2 tablespoons soy oil
1 ounce raisins
1 teaspoon tamari
½ teaspoon cumin
¼ teaspoon salt

Preheat oven to 350 degrees Fahrenheit. Lightly grease a 4 x 8-inch baking dish with soy oil. **Soak** chick peas overnight in 16 ounces water. In the morning, rinse the chick peas, transfer to a saucepan, and add 20 ounces fresh water. **Cook** for 2 hours. **Rinse** dulse 2 or 3 times in cold water to remove sand. **Combine** all ingredients together, and mix well. **Place** in baking dish and bake for 20 minutes.

Serves 2.

Crunchy and Nutty Black Bean Bake

3 ounces black beans
3 ounces cauliflower, cut into bite-size pieces
½ ounce dulse, dry
1½ ounces walnuts
1 ounce raisins
1 ounce carrots, shredded
1 teaspoon minced onion
½ teaspoon salt

Preheat oven to 350 degrees Fahrenheit. Lightly grease a 4 x 8-inch baking dish with soy oil. **Soak** beans overnight in 16 ounces water. In the morning, rinse the beans, transfer to a saucepan, and add 16 ounces fresh water. **Cook** for 1½ hours, or until done. Lightly steam cauliflower for approximately 8 minutes. **Rinse** dulse 2 or 3 times in cold water, and drain. **Combine** all ingredients, and mix well. **Transfer** to baking dish and cover. **Bake** for 20 minutes.

Serves 2.

High-Protein Bean Dip

3 ounces lima beans
3 ounces black beans
4 ounces soy milk
1½ ounces brazil nuts
1 ounce chopped scallions
½ teaspoon coriander
½ teaspoon salt

Soak lima beans overnight in 16 ounces water. Do the same for black beans, separately. In the morning, rinse each bowl of beans, transfer into separate saucepans, and add 16 ounces fresh water to each. **Set** over medium heat for 1½ hours or until soft. **Combine** all ingredients in a blender until smooth. **Serve** cold or at room temperature.

Yields approximately 16 ounces.

Lentil Squash Bake

3 ounces lentils
1½ ounces zucchini
1½ ounces yellow squash
1½ tablespoons soy oil
1 teaspoon minced garlic
½ teaspoon basil
½ teaspoon paprika
½ teaspoon salt
1½ ounces brazil nuts
1 ounce chopped celery

Preheat oven to 375 degrees Fahrenheit. Lightly grease a 4 x 8-inch baking pan with soy oil. **Pour** lentils into a medium saucepan with 12 ounces water. **Set** over medium heat, and cook until tender but not mushy, approximately 30 minutes. **Steam** zucchini and squash. **Combine** zucchini and squash in a blender with oil, garlic, basil, paprika, and salt. **Blend** until smooth. **Combine** lentils with nuts and celery, and toss. **Pour** squash over lentil mixture. **Transfer** to baking pan, and bake for 15 minutes.

Serves 2.

Calcutta Cauliflower

3 ounces cauliflower, cut into

Preheat over to 375 degrees

flowerettes

3 ounces mushrooms, sliced

1 ounce onions, sliced

3 ounces tofu, cut into bite-size
cubes

1½ ounces brazil nuts

2 tablespoons soy oil

½ teaspoon curry powder

½ teaspoon salt

Fahrenheit. Lightly grease a 4 x 8-inch baking dish with soy oil. **Sauté** all ingredients in a skillet with soy oil for 5 minutes over medium heat. **Transfer** to baking dish, and bake for 15 minutes.

Serves 2.

Cauliflower Chick Pea Patties

3 ounces chick peas

3 ounces cauliflower

4½ ounces tofu, cut into bite-size
cubes

2 ounces brazil nuts, chopped

1 tablespoon caraway seeds

1 teaspoon chopped fresh dill

½ teaspoon minced garlic

½ teaspoon salt

⅔ heaping teaspoon arrowroot

4 tablespoons corn oil

Preheat oven to 350 degrees Fahrenheit. Lightly grease a baking sheet with corn oil. **Soak** chick peas overnight in 16 ounces water. In the morning, rinse the beans, transfer to a saucepan, and add 20 ounces fresh water. **Set** over medium heat for 2 hours or until tender.

Steam cauliflower. **Combine** all ingredients in a blender, and blend until coarsely ground. **Transfer** to a bowl, and mix well. **Form** patties with the mixture, and place on baking sheet. **Bake** for 30 minutes or until crispy outside.

Serves 2.

Chick Pea Lentil Patties

3 ounces chick peas

3 ounces lentils

3 ounces carrots, sliced

2 ounces onions, sliced

Preheat oven to 350 degrees Fahrenheit. Lightly grease a baking sheet with corn oil. **Soak** chick peas overnight in 16 ounces water. In the morn-

2 ounces walnuts, chopped
1 teaspoon chopped fresh parsley
½ teaspoon sage
½ teaspoon salt
3 tablespoons corn oil
2 heaping teaspoons arrowroot

ing, rinse the beans, transfer to a saucepan, and add 20 ounces fresh water. **Set** over medium heat for 2 hours or until tender. **Pour** lentils in a medium saucepan with 12 ounces water. **Set** over medium heat, and cook until tender but not mushy, approximately 30 minutes. **Steam** carrots and onions. **Place** all ingredients in a blender, and blend until coarsely ground. **Transfer** to a bowl, and mix well. **Form** patties, and place on baking sheet. **Bake** for 30 minutes or until crispy on outside.

Serves 2.

Nutty Tempeh Burger

1½ ounces barley flour
3 ounces tempeh, cubed
2 ounces brazil nuts, chopped
2 heaping teaspoons Ener-G-Egg Replacer
1 teaspoon minced onion
1 teaspoon minced garlic
½ teaspoon chopped fresh dill
½ teaspoon salt
3 tablespoons corn oil

Preheat oven to 350 degrees Fahrenheit. Lightly grease a baking sheet with corn oil. In a skillet, toast barley flour over medium heat without oil for 5 minutes, stirring occasionally. **Combine** all ingredients in a blender, and blend until coarsely ground. **Transfer** to a bowl, and mix thoroughly. **Form** patties, and place on baking sheet. **Bake** for 20 minutes or until crispy outside.

Serves 2.

Grandma's Lima Bean Soup

3 ounces lima beans
½ ounce dulse, dry
2 ounces carrots, chopped

Soak beans overnight in 3 cups water. In the morning, rinse the beans, transfer to a saucepan, and add

2 ounces onions, chopped
2 ounces celery, chopped
3 tablespoons, soy oil
1 teaspoon fresh, chopped parsley
1 teaspoon salt

4 cups fresh water. **Set** over medium heat with cover for approximately 1½ hours. **Soak** dulse in 8 ounces water. Rinse twice; replace water and drain. After beans have cooked about 1 hour, add dulse, vegetables, and remaining ingredients. **Purée** half this mixture in a blender for 15 seconds until smooth, and add back to soup. Continue cooking for 15 minutes.

Yields approximately 4 cups.

Homemade Mushroom Lentil Soup

3 ounces lentils
3 ounces mushrooms, sliced
3 ounces red cabbage, sliced
1 ounce onion, sliced
3 tablespoons soy oil
½ teaspoon minced garlic
½ teaspoon fresh, chopped dill
½ teaspoon salt

Cook lentils in medium saucepan with 12 ounces water. **Set** over medium heat, and cook until tender but not mushy, about 30 minutes. **Add** remaining ingredients. **Purée** half this mixture in blender for 15 seconds until smooth, and add back to soup. Continue cooking for 20 minutes.

Yields approximately 4 to 5 cups.

Vegetable Black Bean Soup

4½ ounces black beans
3 ounces tofu, cut into bite-size
    cubes
3 ounces parsnip, peeled and sliced
2 ounces celery, sliced
2 ounces carrots, sliced
3 tablespoons soy oil
1 teaspoon mustard
½ teaspoon salt
½ teaspoon tamari

Soak beans overnight in 32 ounces water. In the morning, rinse the beans, transfer to a saucepan, and add 40 ounces fresh water. **Set** over medium heat with cover for approximately 1½ hours. After 1 hour, add remaining ingredients. **Purée** half this mixture in a blender for 15 seconds until smooth. **Add** back to soup. Continue cooking for 15 minutes.

Yields approximately 4 cups.

Caraway Tofu Dip

3 ounces barley
3 ounces tofu
4 tablespoons cider vinegar
4 tablespoons soy oil
1 teaspoon caraway seeds
½ teaspoon mustard
½ teaspoon tamari
¼ teaspoon salt

Cook barley in 16 ounces water. Bring to a boil, then lower to medium heat and cook for 25 minutes. **Place** all ingredients in a blender with 3 ounces water, and purée until smooth.

Yields 14 ounces.

Tempeh Carrot Dip

3 ounces chick peas
1½ ounces tempeh
3 ounces carrots
4 tablespoons soy oil
7 tablespoons cider vinegar
½ teaspoon tamari
½ teaspoon chopped fresh parsley

Soak chick peas overnight in 16 ounces water. In the morning, rinse the beans, transfer to a saucepan, and add 20 ounces fresh water. **Set** over medium heat for 2 hours or until tender. **Steam** tempeh and carrots. **Place** all ingredients in a blender with 3 ounces water, and purée until smooth.

Yields 14 ounces.

Tarragon Bean Dip

3 ounces black beans
3 ounces green beans, cut in half
3 tablespoons corn oil
½ teaspoon tarragon
½ teaspoon salt

Soak beans overnight in 25 ounces water. In the morning, rinse the beans, transfer to a saucepan, and add 36 ounces fresh water. **Set** over medium heat with cover for approximately 1½ hours. **Steam** green beans. **Place** all ingredients in a blender, and purée until smooth.

Yields approximately 11½ ounces.

Fruitful Tofu Pudding

6 ounces pineapple juice
6 ounces banana, sliced
3 ounces nectarine, sliced
3 ounces tofu, cut into bite-size
  cubes
4 ounces barley malt
1 teaspoon vanilla
3 heaping teaspoons Ener-G-Egg
  Replacer
Pinch nutmeg

Place all ingredients in a blender. **Purée** until smooth. **Transfer** to a medium saucepan, and set over medium heat for 5 minutes, stirring frequently. **Chill** for 45 minutes.

Yields 20 ounces.

Golden Blackberry Kanten

12 ounces blackberry juice
2 tablespoons agar-agar
4 ounces banana, sliced
1 ounce golden raisins

Pour juice in a medium saucepan. **Bring** to a boil. **Lower** heat, and agar-agar. **Stir** until agar-agar is dissolved. **Simmer** for 5 minutes. **Chill** in refrigerator until juice begins to gel, around 10 minutes. **Drop** in banana and raisins. **Return** to refrigerator to chill for 1 hour.

Serves 2.

NOTES

Chapter 1

1. Radio interview with Dr. Doris J. Rapp, WBAI-FM, New York City, February 9, 1987.

2. Theron G. Randolph and Ralph W. Moss, *An Alternative Approach to Allergies.* (New York: Bantam, 1982), p. 21.

3. Ibid., pp. 20–21.

4. Claude A. Frazier, *Coping with Food Allergy.* (New York: Time Books, 1974).

5. Rapp, op. cit.

6. Randolph, op. cit., p. 109.

7. Rapp, op. cit.

8. Ibid.

9. Randolph, op. cit., pp. 26–27.

10. Doris J. Rapp, *Allergies and the Hyperactive Child.* (New York: Simon & Schuster, 1979).

11. Rapp, interview, op. cit.

12. Doris J. Rapp, "Environmental Medicine: An Expanded Approach to Allergy," *Buffalo Physician* (February 1986), pp. 16–24.

13. Telephone interview with Dr. Bernard Rimland, November 1986.

14. Roger J. Williams, *Biochemical Individuality.* (New York: John Wiley and Sons, 1956).

15. William H. Philpott, and Dwight K. Kalita, *Brain Allergies: The Psychonutrient Connection.* (New Canaan: Keats, 1980), p. 16.

16. Radio interview with Dr. Doris J. Rapp, WBAI-FM, New York City, August 9, 1983.

Chapter 2

1. Telephone interview with Dr. Theron G. Randolph, February 1987.

2. William H. Philpott and Dwight K. Kalita, *Brain Allergies: The Psychonutrient Connection.* (New Canaan: Keats, 1980), p. 16.

3. Ibid., pp. 17–19.

4. Radio interview with Dr. Doris J. Rapp, WBAI-FM, New York City, February 9, 1987.

5. Radio interview with Jenny Miller, WBAI-FM, New York City, June 8, 1986.

6. Silvano Arieti, ed., *American Handbook on Psychiatry.* (New York: Basic Books, 1953), p. 31.

7. Philpott, op. cit., p. 6.

8. Ibid., p. 5.

9. Radio interview with Dr. Doris J. Rapp, WBAI-FM, New York City, February 9, 1987.

10. Original research, "Iatrogenic Disease," Part I. Penthouse investigative Series, 1984–1987.

11. Telephone interview with Dr. Doris Rapp, March 12, 1987.

12. Ibid.

13. Ibid.

14. Ibid.

15. Ibid.

16. Ibid.

17. Ibid.

18. Ibid.

19. Theron G. Randolph and Ralph W. Moss, *An Alternative Approach to Allergies.* (New York: Bantam, 1982), p. 108.

20. Original research, "Iatrogenic Disease," Part I. Penthouse Investigative Series, 1984–1987.

21. Benjamin Feingold, *Why Your Child Is Hyperactive.* (New York: Random House, 1975).

22. Rapp, interview, op. cit.

23. Randolph, op. cit.

24. Rapp telephone interview, op. cit.

25. Rapp, radio interview, op. cit.

26. Radio interview with Dr. Lendon Smith, WBAI-FM, New York City, April 10, 1987.

27. Alexander Schauss, *Diet, Crime and Delinquency.* (Berkeley: Parker House, 1981), p. 57.

28. William Crook, *Can Your Child Read?, Is He Hyperactive?* (Jackson: Tennessee Professional, 1977).

29. Radio interview with Dr. Steven Schoenthaller, WBAI-FM, New York City, May 15, 1986.

30. Ibid.

31. Schauss, op. cit., p. 11.

32. Ibid.

33. Ibid.

34. Ibid., pp. 11–13.

35. Ibid., p. 14.

36. Philpott, op. cit., p. 16.

37. Schauss, op. cit., p. 19.

38. Ibid., p. 24.

39. Telephone interview with Dr. Steven Schoenthaller, January 1987.

40. Ibid.

41. Ibid.

42. William H. Philpott and Dwight K. Kalita, *Victory Over Diabetes.* (New Canaan: Keats, 1983).

43. Ibid.

44. Editorial, "Can Chocolate Turn You Into a Criminal? . . . Some Experts Say So," *The Wall Street Journal*, June 2, 1977.

45. Ibid.

46. Randolph, op. cit., p. 97.

47. Ibid.

48. Schauss, op. cit.

Chapter 3

1. Claude A. Frazier, *Coping with Food Allergy.* (New York: Times Books, 1974), p. 33.

2. Theron G. Randolph, and Ralph W. Moss, *An Alternative Approach to Allergies.* (New York: Lippincott & Crowell, 1980), p. 123.

3. Albert Rowe, "Allergic Toxemia and Migraine Due to Food Allergy," *California and Western Medicine* 33 (1930): 792.

4. Ibid., p. 788.

5. Ibid., p. 787.

6. Ibid.

7. Ellen C. G. Grant, "Food Allergies and Migraine," *Lancet* (1979):

8. J. Monro, C. Carini, J. Brostoff, et al., "Food Allergy in Migraine," *Lancet* 1(1978): 581.

9. Randolph, op. cit., p. 124.

10. Ellen C. G. Grant, "Oral Contraceptives, Smoking, Migraine and Food Allergy," *Lancet*, 1(1978): 581.

11. Jerome Glaser, "Migraine in Pediatric Practice," *AMA American Journal of Diseases of Children* (1954): 92.

12. Ibid.

13. Ibid., p. 96.

14. Ibid., p. 94.

15. W. E. Nelson, *Textbook of Pediatrics*. (Philadelphia: W. B. Saunders, 1946), p. 1011.

16. J. Egger, J. Wilson, J. F. Soothill, et al., "Is Migraine Food Allergy?" *Lancet* (1983): 865.

17. Ibid., p. 867.

18. Ibid., p. 868.

19. Randolph, op. cit., p. 124.

20. Rowe, op. cit., p. 790.

21. Ibid., p. 785.

22. Ibid.

23. Ibid., p. 793.

24. Theron G. Randolph, "Fatigue and Weakness of Allergic Origin (Allergic Toxemia) to be Differentiated From 'Nervous Fatigue' or Neurasthenia," *Annals of Allergy* 3 (Nov.-Dec. 1945): 418–30.

25. Randolph and Moss, op. cit., p. 14.

26. Frederick Speer, "The Allergic Tension-Fatigue Syndrome," *Pediatric Clinics of North America* 1 (1954): 1029.

27. Frazier, op. cit.

28. Ibid.

29. Albert H. Rowe, "Allergies, Toxemia and Fatigue," *Annals of Allergy* 17 (1959): 9.

30. Randolph and Moss, op. cit.

31. Alan Scott Levin and Merla Zellerbach, *The Type 1 and Type 2 Allergy Relief Program*. (Los Angeles: J. P. Tarcher, 1983), pp. 119–29.

32. Marshall Mandell and Lynne Waller Scanlon, *Dr. Mandell's 5-Day Allergy Relief System*. (Denver: Nutribook, 1979).

33. Marshall Mandell and Anthony Conte, "The Role of Allergy in Arthritis and Rheumatism," *International Academy of Preventive Medicine* 7 (July 1982):

34. *Prevention's New Encyclopedia of Common Diseases*, editors of *Prevention* magazine (Emmaus, Pa.: Rodale Press, 1984), pp. 74–78.

Chapter 4

1. William G. Crook, *The Yeast Connection*. (Jackson, Tenn.: Professional Books, 1986).

2. Radio interview with Dr. Kenneth Cooper, WBAI-FM, New York City, March 20, 1987.

3. Ibid.

4. Theron G. Randolph and Ralph W. Moss, *An Alternative Approach to Allergies*. (New York: Bantam, 1982).

5. Marshall Mandell and Lynne Waller Scanlon, *Dr. Mandell's 5-Day Allergy Relief System* (Denver: Nutribook, 1979), pp. 5–6.

Chapter 5

1. Alan Scott Levin and Merla Zellerbach, *The Type 1 and Type 2 Allergy Relief Program*, (Los Angeles: J. P. Tarcher, 1983), p. 44.

2. Ibid.

3. Theron G. Randolph and Ralph W. Moss, *An Alternative Approach to Allergies*. (New York: Bantam, 1980), p. 161.

4. Laura Stevens, *The Complete Book of Allergy Control*. (New York: Macmillan, 1983), p. 31.

5. Ibid.

6. Radio interview with Dr. Doris J. Rapp, WBAI-FM, New York City, February 9, 1987.

7. Educational videotape prepared by Dr. Doris J. Rapp, January 1987.

8. Ibid.

9. Michael Schachter, David Scheinkin, and Richard Hutton, *Food, Mind and Mood.* (New York: Warner Books, 1977), pp. 115–17.

10. Marshall Mandell and Lynne Waller Scanlon, *Dr. Mandell's 5-Day Allergy Relief System.* (Denver: Nutribook, 1979), p. 248.

11. Schachter et al., op. cit., pp. 73, 101–102.

12. Doris Rapp, *Allergies and Your Family.* (New York: Sterling Publishers, 1981), p. 146.

13. Sharon Faelton, *The Allergy Self-Help Book.* (Emmaus, Pa.: Rodale Press, 1983), p. 189.

14. Doris Rapp, *Allergies and the Hyperactive Child.* (New York: Simon & Schuster, 1979), pp. 88–89.

Chapter 6

1. Gary Null and Leonard Steinman, "Natural Healers: A Reborn Medical Therapy," *Penthouse*, May 1986, p. 136.

2. Ibid.

3. Ibid, p. 136–37. See also Harris L. Coulter's *Divided Legacy* (Richmond, CA: North Atlantic Books, 1982).

4. Ibid. p. 137.

5. Ibid.
6. Ibid. p. 112.
7. Ibid. p. 138.
8. Ibid.
9. Ibid.
10. Radio interview with Dr. Richard Podell, WBAI-FM, New York City, February 6, 1987.
11. Ibid.
12. Linus Pauling, *How to Live Longer and Feel Better*. (New York: W. H. Freeman, 1986), pp. 231–32.
13. Ibid., pp. 173–74.
14. Ibid. pp. 175–76.
15. Radio interview with Dr. Doris J. Rapp, WBAI-FM, New York, February 9, 1987.
16. Theron G. Randolph and Ralph W. Moss, *An Alternative Approach to Allergies*. (New York: Bantam Books, 1982).
19. Podell, op. cit.
20. Randolph and Moss, op. cit.
21. Ibid.
22. Radio interview with Dr. Lendon Smith, WBAI-FM, New York City, April 10, 1987.
23. W. Bullock, C. Deamer, O. L. Frick, et al., Letters to the Editor, *Pediatrics* 46 (1970): 971.
24. Radio interview with Dr. Marshall Mandell, WBAI-FM, New York City, March 15, 1987.
25. American Academy of Allergy and Immunology Committee on Adverse Reactions to Foods, National Institutes of Health (Washington, D.C.: U.S. Government Printing Office, 1984).
26. Podell, op. cit.
27. Ibid.
28. Mandell, op. cit.
29. William H. Philpott and Dwight K. Kalita, *Brain Allergies: The Psychonutrient Connection*. (New Canaan: Keats, 1980).
30. Rapp, op. cit.
31. William G. Crook, *Are You Allergic?* (Jackson, Tenn.: Professional Books, 1978).
32. Ibid.
33. Rapp, op. cit.
34. Philpott, op. cit., p. 8.

Chapter 7
1. Radio interview with Dr. John McDougall, WBAI-FM, New York City, March 3, 1987.
2. Ibid.
3. Hara Marano, "The Problem with Protein," *New York*, March 5, 1979, p. 50.
4. Ibid.
5. McDougall, op. cit.
6. Frances Moore Lappé, *Diet for a Small Planet*. (New York: Ballantine, 1982).
7. Robert Goodhart and Maurice Shils, *Modern Nutrition in Health and Disease*.

Philadelphia: Lea and Febiger, 1980, p. 91.

8. McDougall, op. cit.

9. Marano, op. cit.

10. *Gary Null's Natural Living Newsletter*, "Dangerous Chemicals in Meat", no. 40.

11. McDougall, op. cit.

12. Gary Null, *The Egg Project*, 1984.

13. Ibid.

BIBLIOGRAPHY

Crook, William G. *The Yeast Connection.* 3d ed. (Jackson, Tenn.: Professional Books, 1986).

Faelten, Sharon. *The Allergy Self-Help Book.* (Emmaus, Pa.: Rodale, 1983).

Feingold, Benjamin. *Why Your Child Is Hyperactive.* (New York: Random House, 1975).

Levin, Alan Scott, and Merla Zellerbach. *The Type 1 and Type 2 Allergy Relief Program.* (Los Angeles: J.P. Tarcher, 1983).

Mandell, Marshall. *Dr. Mandell's Lifetime Arthritis Relief System.* (New York: Berkeley, 1983).

Mandell, Marshall, and Lynne Waller Scanlon. *Dr. Mandell's 5-Day Allergy Relief System.* (Denver: Nutribook, 1979).

Null, Gary. *The Complete Guide to Health and Nutrition.* (New York: Dell Publishing, 1984).

Randolph, Theron G., and Ralph W. Moss. *An Alternative Approach to Allergies.* (New York: Harper and Row, 1981).

Rapp, Doris J. *Allergies and the Hyperactive Child.* (New York: Simon and Schuster, 1979).

Rapp, Doris J. *Allergies and Your Family.* (New York: Sterling, 1981).

Scheinkin, David, Michael Schacter, and Richard Hutton. *Food, Mind and Mood.* (New York: Warner Books, 1979).

Stevens, Laura. *The Complete Book of Allergy Control.* (New York: Macmillan, 1983).

Index